ESTROGEN

ESTROGEN

HOW AND WHY IT CAN SAVE YOUR LIFE

ADAM ROMOFF, M.D.
with INA YALOF

Golden Books
New York

Golden Books®
888 Seventh Avenue
New York, NY 10106

Designed by Stanley S. Drate/Folio Graphics Co. Inc.

Manufactured in the United States of America

10 9 8 7 6 5 4 3 2 1

Library of Congress Cataloging-in-Publication Data

Romoff, Adam.
Estrogen : how and why it can save your life / Adam Romoff, with Ina Yalof.
p. cm.
Includes bibliographical references and index.
ISBN 1-58238-012-0 (alk. paper)
1. Estrogen—Therapeutic use—Side effects. 2. Menopause—Hormone therapy. 3. Therapeutics—Complications. I. Yalof, Ina. II. Title.
RG186.R65 1999
615′.366—dc21 98-31174
CIP

To my wife, Vivien,
with whom my soul is linked forever.

CONTENTS

INTRODUCTION

Most menopausal women are not taking estrogen. By choosing not to take this hormone, these women are giving up the natural advantage estrogen bestows upon them without a fight. As a result, tens of thousands of precious lives are being lost each year in the United States alone.

It has been my privilege to practice and teach obstetrics and gynecology over the past twenty years. Over that time, as brilliant scientific research has revealed the nature of estrogen's effects on the body, I have become convinced that estrogen saves lives. In my practice, however, I have been dismayed at how difficult it is for many of my patients to become comfortable with the notion of taking hormone replacement. It is for that reason that I have written this book.

Ultimately, I believe, the weight of the evidence supporting estrogen use will overcome women's deeply rooted fears and ambivalence, so that it will become the norm sometime in the next century. My concern is that this process will be devastatingly slow. It is my fervent hope to save lives by hastening the process of acceptance—in the most honest and simple terms—by trying to convince *you* to take estrogen—now, in this century.

It's a formidable task. Everybody is afraid of breast cancer. This fear is the most common reason why women discontinue or never begin hormone-replacement therapy.

In the course of this book, I will discuss the results of numerous studies revealing that estrogen use causes *no* increase in breast cancer in the first five years of use, and *possibly* only a small, clinically insignificant increase with long-term use.

In my personal judgment, estrogen causes *no* increase in deaths from breast cancer. Even if there is a small increase in the occurrence of breast cancer with long-term use of estrogen, it is *overwhelmed* by estrogen's profoundly large benefit, its life-saving protection against heart disease, which is 5 to 10 times more likely to affect you than is breast cancer.

"The problem," as was recently expressed to me by one learned professor (also employed as a part-time consultant for Evista, the new "designer" estrogen), "is that you can talk to women about heart disease until you are blue in the face. All they care about is breast cancer . . . and maybe osteoporosis is getting a little play." Unfortunately, I'm afraid that the professor-salesman is probably correct. But I have an even greater fear of his solution, which is to offer women an unproven, probably third-rate, flash-in-the-pan estrogen substitute. These are the very women whose fears of breast and uterine cancer, misgivings about side effects, and overall distrust of estrogen have led them to refuse it in the first place.

I will discuss the new estrogens in some detail later, but I want to state here unequivocally that I believe the widespread use of any "designer" estrogen without proof of its ability to protect against heart disease can cost untold loss of life—even if some degree of protection against breast cancer is provided.

In my opinion, the unrestrained and irresponsible proclamation of promises—that a designer estrogen will do everything you ever wanted without worry, or that eating *soy muffins* is a way to hormonal health—threatens to further distort the vision of women faced with crucial decisions about their health and lives. Fully one-third of those lives will be spent in the postmenopausal years. So there is an urgent need to provide women with information unfettered by hidden bias or hidden agenda.

Given my strong feelings about these issues, my presentation will have an undeniable slant. Nonetheless, I hope to provide you with a broad base of scientific knowledge that will enable you to join us in the medical profession as we seek to preserve life.

Through the Looking Glass: Our Backward Perception of Breast Cancer and Heart Disease

The reality is, while roughly 46,000 women die of breast cancer each year in the United States, about 500,000 die from cardiovascular disease. There is no controversy about these numbers. How they are *perceived*, however, is something else altogether. In a recent Gallup poll, about 40 percent of women said they thought they were going to die from breast cancer. This proportion is *ten times* higher than the actual chance of about 4 percent. Only about 10 percent of women listed heart disease as their primary concern when in fact, *almost half* of women will eventually die from cardiovascular disease.

Without trying to remember them, read the following numbers to get a sense of their weight relative to one another: Women have about a 23 percent chance of dying from coronary-artery disease, in contrast to only 4 percent from breast cancer, 2.5 percent from bone fractures/osteoporosis and 2 percent from cancers of the reproductive tract.

Before I continue, I must acknowledge that here we are leaving the world of fact and entering the world of probability. However, this is the world of clinical medicine. It is in this context that the following premise emerges: *Estrogen most probably reduces the chance of death from cardiovascular disease by one-half, and in so doing represents the potential to save an extraordinary number of lives.*

How Is It Possible that Estrogen Can Save So Many Lives?

In 1994, Dr. Robin Gorsky and her colleagues wrote an article that I haven't been able to stop thinking about. In her article, Dr. Gorsky made various presumptions about estrogen's risks and benefits based upon the available scientific data, and then analyzed the potential outcome of two groups of women. One group included 10,000 women who took estrogen from age fifty to age seventy-five. The other group included 10,000 women who did *not* take hormones.

Results of the study showed that at age seventy-five, of the 10,000 women who took estrogen, 567 lives were saved from heart disease, 75 lives were saved from complications due to hip fracture, and 39 lives were lost to breast cancer. (I do *not* include here 29 lives cited that were lost to uterine cancer because today, with the modern use of progesterone, this would almost certainly not be the case.)

This represents 642 lives saved versus 39 lives lost.

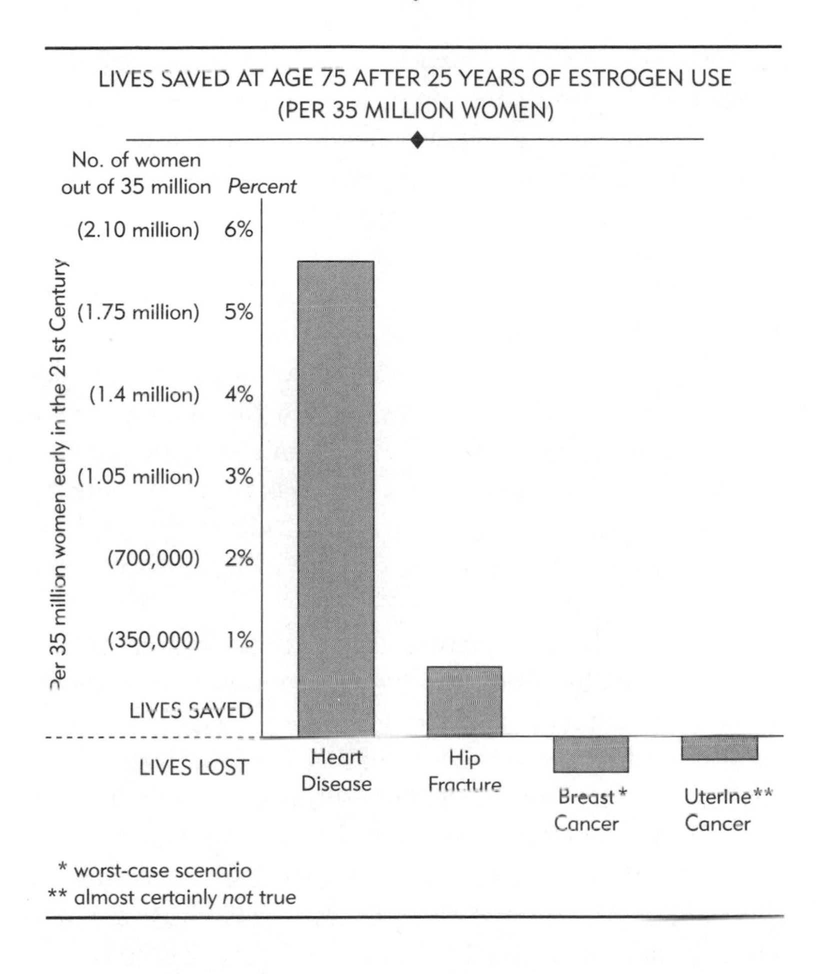

This suggests that the lives of some 600 women out of every 10,000 could be saved.

This is a *6 percent* survival advantage.

In a population of 35 million women taking estrogen for twenty-five years from age fifty to age seventy-five, as could occur early in the next century, a 6 percent survival advantage provided by estrogen use would enable an additional *2.1 million* women to reach age seventy-five.

Two million lives over twenty-five years translates into

tens of thousands of lives each year. Right now, based on current U.S. population data, I estimate that *20,000 to 60,000 preventable, premature deaths of women are occurring each year because only 15 percent to 30 percent of postmenopausal women take estrogen long term.* This is a modern-day tragedy.

Frankly, when faced with the calculation of such an overwhelming loss of life, along with the fact that you seem to be the only one who recognizes it, the inescapable conclusion you come to is that *you must be wrong.* This is especially true when virtually every medical publication suggests that we must assess the risks and benefits of hormone-replacement therapy on an individualized basis, implying that there are, indeed, many women who should *not* take estrogen.

However, I subsequently found that calculations by other responsible investigators were consistent with the findings of Dr. Gorsky.* So I think I'm right. One can quibble with the simplistic calculations and argue about the *degree* of cardioprotection and the risks of breast cancer and uterine cancer, but the numbers speak for themselves. Furthermore, as we continue to learn about the effects of estrogen on the heart, blood vessels, brain, and bone tissue, estrogen's life-enhancing and preserving effects will certainly seem logical, if not miraculous.

Why Aren't More Women Taking Estrogen?

Most estimates place the proportion of menopausal and postmenopausal women taking estrogen as varying from

*These studies are noted in Appendix A.

1 in 6 to 1 in 4. This is probably true overall, even though there are some geographic areas where the use of estrogen-replacement therapy is more common. So why are so few women enjoying the benefits of estrogen?

Nobody knows for sure. Historically, estrogen's path seemed quite smooth in the 1960s. This was particularly evident after publication in 1966 of the highly popular *Feminine Forever,* a book by Dr. Robert Wilson that fed into women's desire for youth, attractiveness, and relief from menopausal symptoms. As many of you may remember, what followed was a sea change in the social, political, and medical landscapes. By the 1970s, two highly charged medical issues became apparent. First, estrogen use was found to cause increased risk of uterine cancer (at that time, protective progesterone was not routinely added), and second, high-dose birth control pills were found to cause an increased incidence of blood-clot formation.

Understandably, doubts about the quality of research pertaining to women's health—and, indeed, doubts about the treatment of women by the predominately male medical profession—abounded. All this took place at around the same time feminism and the sexual revolution were fast becoming integrated into the American culture. What resulted were distrustful and at best highly conflicted feelings about estrogen. Most women simply stopped taking it.

In the decades since then, our health-consciousness has increased significantly. While this trend has been accompanied by a great many positive changes, increased use of estrogen is unfortunately not one of them. There are probably three major reasons for this: the continued fear of breast and uterine cancer, misgivings about estrogen's side effects, and the sense that women feel they "don't need it."

As women's awareness of estrogen's life-enhancing benefits increases, and their fears of breast cancer are allayed by scientific information, perhaps side effects such as bleeding and breast tenderness will become easier to tolerate. In essence, if women fully understand the *need* for hormone replacement, any possible discomfort from side effects will *not* be perceived as a problem, and estrogen use will ultimately become the norm.

One can only hope.

The Increasing Importance of the Menopausal Years: A Mandate for the Future

"So what did they do *before* estrogen was invented?" is a question often voiced in my office by exasperated and ambivalent patients seeking a solution to their concerns.

To begin with, people usually didn't *live* past fifty until the turn of the century. In the Victorian era, the life expectancy was about age forty-five. During the Roman Empire, people lived only until they were about twenty-five years old! Yet the age of menopause—roughly around fifty—is thought to have remained relatively stable over time. This means that on average, before the turn of the century, before the concept of estrogen replacement, most women died before they ever reached menopause.

Today, though the biological limit of life is not increasing, life *expectancy* is. Look at what has happened in the twentieth century alone. A woman born in 1990 had a life expectancy of seventy-nine years. If she lived to her sixty-fifth birthday, she could expect to live until just shy of her eighty-fifth birthday. By 2050, life expectancy will be about eighty-four years, and sixty-five-year-olds can expect to survive until age eighty-eight—forty or so years *beyond* the onset of menopause. This dramatic increase in life expectancy is essentially due to scientific and medical progress (which, I notice, never seems to get any credit for being "natural"). As Dr. Charles Hammond of Duke University states: "That we will eventually die is certain. What we hope to do is postpone illness and compress morbidity. We would live relatively healthy and long lives, then compress our illnesses into a short period of time just before our deaths at about the age of eighty-five. Ideally, disease is something not treated but prevented or postponed."

Early in the next century, 1 person in 5 will be older than sixty-five. Women will spend more than one-third of their lives after menopause. By preventing and delaying the ravages of heart disease, Alzheimer's disease, and osteoporosis, as well as providing beneficial effects on memory and cognition, hormone-replacement therapy also stands to prevent premature deaths and extend the quality of life. Knowledge and information about estrogen—communicated without hidden agenda or bias and without the simplistic "sound bite" approach that has infused our popular culture—is vital. Women's lives depend on it.

1

DECREASING THE FEAR OF BREAST CANCER:

A First Step

The extraordinary fear of breast cancer deters tragically large numbers of women from taking estrogen. However, recent scientific studies reveal that using estrogen in doses that protect against heart disease, osteoporosis, and probably Alzheimer's disease does *not* significantly increase the risk of developing breast cancer.

In fact, we can now say with confidence that taking estrogen for *up to five years* does *not* cause breast cancer. Still, lingering doubt remains as to whether long-term use (for more than five years) *might* cause a small increase in the risk of developing the disease. As we shall see, the data are by no means persuasive. In fact, two vitally important perspectives are strikingly clear:

- If estrogen had *any* strong effect on the occurrence of breast cancer, good *or* bad, it would have been discovered long ago—and certainly by now.

- The profoundly *large* and *proven* life-preserving benefits of estrogen *overwhelm* estrogen's *small*, and as yet *unproven*, negative effect on breast cancer.

With every ounce of my professional integrity, I believe this to be true.

Dealing with Fear: Toward a Clearer Perspective

In the introduction I discussed a recent Gallup poll in which women were asked what they thought they were going to die from. Their responses were so startling, they merit being repeated. *Forty percent* of the women believed they were going to die from breast cancer. This is *ten times* higher than the accepted truth, which is that *4 percent* of women die from breast cancer. In fact, more than 40 percent of women will die from *cardiovascular disease*, not breast cancer. And yet only 10 percent of the women polled listed that as their primary concern.

Take a look at the bar graph on the next page. Understand that it represents widely accepted medical fact about which there is no controversy, and burn it into your brain.

Remember this picture. Everybody—patients and doctors, myself included—forgets the numbers. This graph represents the relative impact of various disease states on life and death. Notice that cardiovascular disease kills women at a rate ten times higher than breast cancer.

Please don't misunderstand me. I am not in any way minimizing the breast cancer issue. I am simply trying to put things into perspective. Because cardiovascular disease is so much more prevalent than breast cancer, *any* protective effect against heart disease will save far more lives than might be lost from any increase in breast cancer.

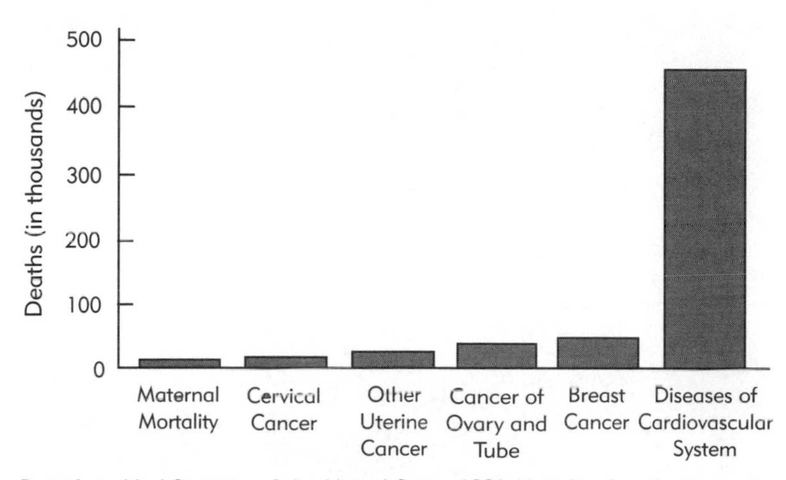

Data from *Vital Statistics of the United States 1981 Mortality, Part A*, Hyattsville, Maryland: National Center for Health Statistics, 1986.

Breast cancer is the most common site (32 percent of all cases) of cancer in women. About 180,000 cases occur in the United States each year. Some 46,000 women die from breast cancer each year, reflecting a mortality rate that has been largely unchanged since 1940. The good news is, five-year survival for localized breast cancer has risen from 78 percent in the 1940s to 94 percent in 1995. This has been attributed to earlier diagnosis resulting from the increased use of high-resolution mammography, and a surge in programs educating women about the disease—both significant lifesavers.

Over the past four years, with more cases being diagnosed earlier, we are finally seeing a drop in the overall mortality rate for breast cancer. On another positive note, about two-thirds of all women with breast cancer will become long-term survivors.

Breast cancer incidence increases with age. However, as you can see, the 1 in 8, or 1 in 9, risk of developing the disease occurs only if you live to be about eighty-five or

THE CHANCES OF DEVELOPING BREAST CANCER ACCORDING TO AGE

By age 25	1 in 19,608
By age 30	1 in 2,525
By age 35	1 in 622
By age 40	1 in 217
By age 45	1 in 93
By age 50	1 in 50
By age 55	1 in 33
By age 60	1 in 24
By age 65	1 in 17
By age 70	1 in 14
By age 75	1 in 11
By age 80	1 in 10
By age 85	1 in 9
Lifetime	1 in 8

Data from Feuer, E.J., et al, "The Lifetime Risk of Developing Breast Cancer," *Journal of the National Cancer Institute*, 85: 892, 1993.

ninety years old. So it's *not quite* true that "every woman has a 1 in 8 chance of developing breast cancer."

Alas, what is true is that, of malignancies, *lung cancer, not breast cancer*, has become the leading cause of cancer deaths in women—a fact I attribute entirely to social change and the power of Madison Avenue. The Virginia Slims ad campaign attaching cigarette smoking to the legitimate feminist concerns of women was perhaps the most pernicious in history—as witness the meteoric rise of lung cancer over the past two decades.

Life is precious. If we let the fear of breast cancer cloud our vision and distort our judgment, we run the risk of making the wrong decisions, particularly regarding the life-saving capabilities of estrogen. So when daily

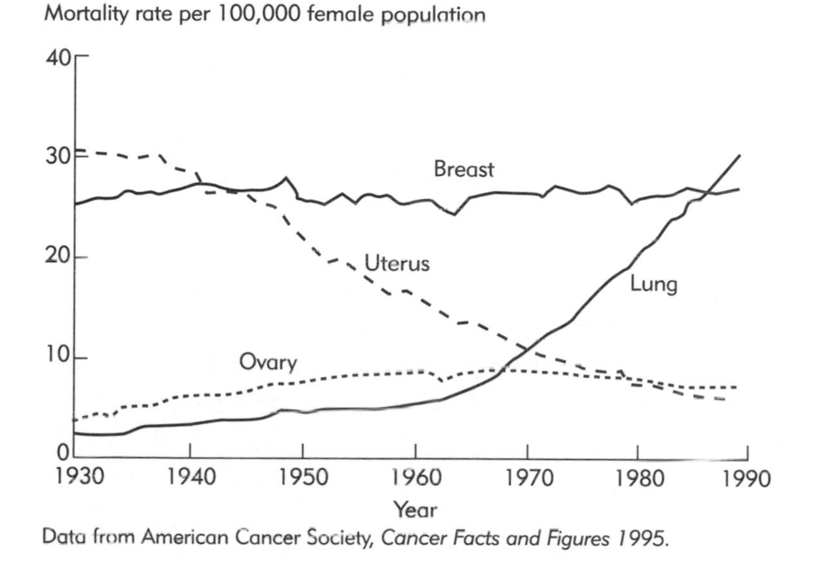

Data from American Cancer Society, *Cancer Facts and Figures 1995.*

headlines tweak our fears and play with our emotions, we must remember the larger picture.

An Approach to the Information

In the medical community, arguments abound over conflicting data and theory concerning estrogen's connection to breast cancer. Ironically, there is probably more agreement about the ultimate conclusion—that estrogen use *does not* have any large effect on the occurrence of breast cancer—than there is about the supporting details. Watching all of this debate is an uneasy public. So on the one side we have the researchers, who are a bit edgy about whether or not their data are fairly presented. On the other side are the heightened concerns and frayed nerve endings of a doubtful public. At times I have found any attempt to navigate these difficult waters virtually impossible.

As we begin to explore the art and science of breast cancer research as it relates to estrogen, I have necessarily had to make a great many value judgments. These judgments, especially in the face of incomplete data, are certainly subject to bias and error. Still, I hope to provide a reliable foundation upon which you can build your own knowledge, just as we in medicine build ours.

The information that follows is based on medical texts and published research studies selected from the medical literature. The sources for each study cited can be found in the bibliography of this book. The interested reader is by all means encouraged to obtain and read the studies herself and to make her own personal assessment of the data.

Let's take an in-depth look at breast cancer as it relates first to a woman's own hormones (estrogen and progesterone) and, second, to estrogen replacement after menopause. We will also reappraise the use of estrogen in breast cancer survivors.

The Effect of a Woman's Own Hormones on Breast Cancer

ESTROGEN

The fundamental logic that estrogen plays a role in promoting breast cancer at some point in a woman's life is based in part on the following facts:

- Breast cancer is 100 times more common in women than in men.
- Breast cancer always occurs after puberty, when estrogen is first produced.
- Breast cancer cells contain estrogen receptors which are biologically active.

The relative effect of a woman's own estrogen on her chances of getting breast cancer may be related to the *type* of estrogen she secretes. Women manufacture essentially three types of estrogen: estradiol, estrone, and estriol. Estradiol is the most potent form and it alone is often called "natural" estrogen. Estrone is weaker and estriol is the weakest of the three.

Women who have had early pregnancies subsequently create a hormonal environment with higher levels of the weaker estriol—which might block some of the effects of the more potent estrogens, estradiol and estrone. This may be one mechanism by which early pregnancy provides protection against breast cancer.

Also of note is that premenopausal Asian women have a lower incidence of breast cancer but *more* estriol than Caucasian women. But when these women migrate to the United States, their breast-cancer rate increases and their estriol decreases. Why this happens is not fully understood (some scientists believe it is diet-related) but it underscores the notion that when hormones are replaced, it is important to consider the *type* of estrogen prescribed.

Another aspect concerns the *balance* in a woman's body between her own estrogen and progesterone. It has been theorized that the prolonged presence of estrogen *without* progesterone makes breast cells more susceptible to outside environmental carcinogens.

Consequently, any period in a woman's life when she has levels of estrogen that are not "opposed" or balanced by progesterone might provide a window of opportunity for carcinogens to interact with susceptible breast tissues—beginning a malignant process which may not become apparent until years later. This has been called the Estrogen Window Hypothesis, as proposed by Dr. Stanley Korenman.

One such "window" occurs during puberty, when estrogen production has started but regular periods (with their balancing progesterone) have not yet begun. In other words, a window of estrogen-only environment opens in puberty, but is closed when a woman begins to ovulate or has a first pregnancy—both of which produce high levels of progesterone.

Supporting this notion are data showing that women who do not ovulate, start to menstruate at a younger age, have a late menopause, or delay their first pregnancy have a wider "estrogen window" and may therefore be viewed as having an increased risk of breast cancer. It should be pointed out that these theories, while attractive, have *not* been conclusively proven by scientific studies.

PROGESTERONE

During each normal menstrual cycle, a woman ovulates and produces progesterone for about two weeks. It is during these two weeks, under the dominant influence of progesterone, that breast cells grow and divide. This sole fact provides the logical underpinning for an opposing hypothesis that *progesterone* may be the key initiator of breast cancer.

But here, too, the data are conflicting and unconvincing. In some laboratory experiments, breast cancer cells are *stimulated* by progesterone; in others, they are *inhibited* by it. In fact, studies of normal breast cells reveal that progestins inhibit growth. Further, women who ultimately develop breast cancer do not have different blood levels of progesterone than those who do not.

Try as they might, researchers have not been able to identify a particular hormonal profile—that is, a particular combination of estrogen and progesterone levels unique to women who develop breast cancer.

Resolving the Paradox: Considering that Estrogen May Not *Be Dangerous*

You cannot avoid the following logic: Women have estrogen; men have very little. Women get breast cancer; men rarely do. There *has* to be a link, a degree of danger in the use of estrogen. So if someone says, "Estrogen has little connection to breast cancer," it *can't* be true. Yet it probably *is*. Hence, the paradox.

As much as we all (doctors and patients alike) try to reassure ourselves, the problem lies in the fact that no one fully understands the biology, the genetics, or the behavior of the molecules that determine the difference between benign and malignant cells. Rather, at this point we know only what we see—what we can observe.

The following observations are based on scientific studies and provide reassurance that estrogen and progesterone, as they relate to breast cancer, may indeed be safe.

PREGNANCY AND BREAST CANCER

Despite the very high levels of estrogen and progesterone secreted during pregnancy, there is *no* difference in survival between women who are pregnant and those who aren't when they are matched for age and stage of disease. (It is possible, however, that difficulty examining a pregnant woman's breasts may result in pregnant women being diagnosed at a more advanced stage of disease.) In those women who have had breast cancer previously diagnosed and treated, subsequent pregnancy appears to have *no* negative effect on survival.

BIRTH-CONTROL PILLS AND BREAST CANCER

Birth-control pills contain doses of estrogen and progestin about two to four times higher than those used in hormone-replacement therapy. And yet, there is *no* significant negative effect on breast cells from the use of birth-control pills.

Though some controversy remains, we should allow these observations about pregnancy and birth-control pills, both of which result in or contain higher-than-normal estrogen levels, to reassure us about at least the *plausibility* of the theory that *estrogen is not dangerous.*

Estrogen-Replacement Therapy and Breast Cancer

Large and comprehensive studies show "short term" use of estrogen—that is, estrogen use for up to five years—with or without progestin, has no effect at all on the risk of developing breast cancer. However, if you wish to partake fully of estrogen's life-preserving benefits to the heart, bones, and brain, you must elect "long term" use of estrogen.

Some studies show *no* increase at all in the occurrence of breast cancer with the long-term use of estrogen. Other studies show a small increased risk. Each highly experienced researcher seems to have his or her individual opinion about what the truth is. *What experts do agree about is that if there is any increase in the occurrence of breast cancer associated with the long-term use of estrogen, it is small.*

One of the terms used in epidemiological research that

you will hear over and over again is "relative risk."* It works like this: Everybody starts out with the same basic risk of getting a disease. That risk is 1. If something you do, let's say eating animal fat, *doubles* your risk of getting that disease, then your relative risk is increased to 2. If eating animal fat triples your risk, your relative risk is 3, and so on. Conversely, if eating vegetables cuts in half the chances of getting the disease, people who eat vegetables have a relative risk of 0.5 for that disease. When scientists evaluate a degree of danger, they generally take note of a relative risk of 2 or higher.

In the past, when unopposed estrogen was used (estrogen without progesterone added to protect the uterus), the incidence of early uterine cancer was *consistently* high. The numbers, depending on whose study you are citing, ranged from four to ten times higher. These relative risks of 4 to 10 present the kind of data researchers feel confident about.

Contrast this to the data on long-term use of estrogen and breast cancer. The data are *not* consistent. The relative risk ranges from 1 (*no* effect) to about 1.4 (at most a *small* effect, and nowhere near the higher numbers seen with unopposed estrogen and uterine cancer). In this case, scientists are *not* comfortable making any predictions regarding the long-term use of estrogen as it relates to breast cancer except to say that, if there is any effect at all, it is small and may not be clinically significant.

With this overview in mind, let's look at the results of some of the recent and ongoing studies.

*For a more complete discussion of relative versus absolute risk, refer to Appendix B.

The Studies

THE CANCER AND SEX HORMONE STUDY

In 1987, the Centers for Disease Control found *no* increased risk of breast cancer in postmenopausal women using estrogen. The duration of therapy (up to 20 years or longer) had *no* effect, nor did a positive family history of breast cancer or previous benign breast disease.

NURSES HEALTH STUDY

This study, which we will cite throughout this book, has been following 120,000 women, all nurses, for more than twenty years. The women provided information every two years regarding, among other things, their use of hormones. About 30 percent of the women are current users, 30 percent are past users, and 40 percent never used hormones. The results of sixteen years of follow-up (1976 to 1992) were reported in 1995. *No* link to breast cancer was found for any group of women using estrogen five years or less. Similarly, women who used estrogen long term in the past had no increased risk. However, one group of women, *current long-term* users, did show an increased risk of developing breast cancer and an increased risk of breast cancer mortality (also a relative risk of about 1.4).

This ongoing study is quite large and no critical analysis can completely nullify these last results. Nonetheless, the following considerations challenge the above findings:

- Most other studies have found a 15 to 20 percent *decreased* risk of breast cancer mortality among estrogen users. The large Leisure World Study reported a 19 percent decreased breast cancer mortality rate in estrogen users, although the women in this study may have benefited from the increased use of mammography. This is called a "surveillance bias."

- The risk of breast cancer increases with age. Because many estrogen users survive longer than women who have never used estrogen, the estrogen users may have a slightly higher occurrence of breast cancer *simply because they live longer.* It is altogether possible that women who don't take estrogen may die of cardiovascular disease before they ever have a chance to contract breast cancer. This is called "prevalence bias."
- Past users and current long-term users may be different from one another in terms of other risk factors and characteristics.
- As was previously noted, a relative risk of 1.4 is small and does not inspire confidence among sophisticated researchers.

AMERICAN CANCER SOCIETY STUDY

This study followed more than 400,000 postmenopausal women from 1982 to 1991. At enrollment, the women were asked whether they were using estrogen replacement (although there is no information collected as to how long they continued it). The women who used estrogen had a 16 percent *reduction* in risk for breast cancer mortality.

THE NATIONAL CANCER INSTITUTE'S BREAST CANCER DETECTION STUDY

No increase in breast cancer risk was shown in women who took estrogen. One group of hormone users did have a small increased relative risk of 1.2, but analysis by the researchers showed that this was *not* statistically significant.

ADDITIONAL STUDIES

Two large studies from the Eastern United States and Toronto, Canada, showed *no* increased risk for up to fifteen years of estrogen use.

A study from the state of Washington found *no* increased risk of breast cancer with either past or current use of estrogen, with or without progestin.

One study by Dupont involved 10,000 women who had breast biopsies for benign disease. The study showed that estrogen use in these women did *not* increase the risk of breast cancer. In fact, *estrogen users who had precancerous cells on their biopsies actually had a reduction in risk of breast cancer.*

Trying to Look at Everything: The Technique of Meta-Analysis

Clearly, one can always pick and choose from among the many different studies to make a point. For example, concerning the results of estrogen's effect on breast cancer, there are some small studies that show a larger increased risk, and other small studies that show a considerably reduced risk. Due to the modest size of the studies, their outcomes are less powerful and can be less accurate than the larger studies. In an attempt to make better sense of the conflicting data, scientists sometimes try to "add up the numbers" of all the previous studies, large and small, to see what result emerges. This technique is called meta-analysis. Information gathered by this method can be thought-provoking and quite revealing.

Let me first point out, however, some difficulties with this technique, especially as it relates to estrogen and breast cancer.

- The studies in question used different *doses* and *types* of estrogen and progestin.
- The studies used different methods. Some studies gave women estrogen and then looked forward in time to see if the women developed breast cancer. Other studies began with patients who had breast cancer and looked backward to see what percentage of these women took estrogen. Each of these methods has its own particular problems and biases.
- The studies occurred during different decades and with the varying use of technology available at the time.
- The author of any meta-analysis may have his or her own bias as to whether a study should be included or not.

Some leading researchers are of the opinion that adding together different studies doesn't make these problems and biases go away but instead can actually *magnify* them. Nonetheless, meta-analysis is firmly established as a way to evaluate scientific data. The following are highlights of some current studies.

- In 1988, an Australian study by Armstrong entitled "Oestrogen Therapy After the Menopause—Boon or Bain?" looked at twenty-three studies and stated "unequivocally" that conjugated estrogen (Premarin) use at a standard low dose of 0.625 mg did not increase breast cancer risk.

- In their 1991 meta-analysis, Dupont and Page found *no* increased risk with 0.625 mg of conjugated estrogen (Premarin) used for any length of time. They raised the question as to whether the higher dose of 1.25 mg caused a small increase in breast cancer incidence, but determined it was not statistically significant.
- In 1992 the Centers for Disease Control (CDC) in Atlanta published an analysis of the literature and concluded that there was *no* increased risk associated with up to five years of estrogen use. However, the long-term use of estrogen (defined by the authors as more than fifteen years of use) was associated with a small increased risk (relative risk 1.3). This was also the *only* meta-analysis to find a link between a family history of breast cancer and an enhanced risk from estrogen use.
- In 1992, Solero-Arenas and other researchers from Spain found a very slight (relative risk 1.1) increased risk overall among estrogen users. However, in one subgroup, the use of 0.625 mg of conjugated estrogen was not associated with any increased risk.
- The authors of the Nurses Health Study found no increased risk in the women who "ever" used estrogen. This refers to women who used estrogen at any time in their lives and may or may not have stopped using it. This was the strongest finding of the study. However, as noted, much weaker data supported the finding of a small increased risk among current long-term users. The dose of estrogen used had no effect on the risk.

The Nachtigall Study and The Women's Health Initiative

Lila Nachtigall, M.D., a highly respected clinician, teacher, and researcher, conducted the only significant randomized trial to date of hormone use and the development of breast cancer. Beginning in 1965, Nachtigall placed one group of women on estrogen-progestin therapy. Another group received no treatment. Each woman who received treatment was "matched" for age and health status to a woman who did not receive treatment. This statistical technique is called a matched-pairs analysis.

After ten years, the women *chose* whether they wanted to stop or to continue treatment, and the study continued for another twelve years. Also at the ten-year point, the dose was decreased from 2.5 mg of Premarin (a very high dose, we now know) to the lower dose of 0.625 mg.

During the entire twenty-two years of the study, *no* breast cancer developed in the 116 women who received hormone-replacement therapy, but breast cancers were found in 6 of the 52 women who did not take it. The numbers of women involved in this study are small, but the results are statistically significant. When such small numbers are involved, the results can always turn out to be a chance finding or subject to other error. Nonetheless, this is the only *completed* study of its kind to date.

There is currently a large, ongoing study in the United States—The Women's Health Initiative—that will attempt to reproduce these methods. This study will eventually include tens of thousands of women, half of whom won't take estrogen. Who takes estrogen and who doesn't is currently being decided by random selection, *not* by choice.

If one can get past the subliminal hype of the study's name—Women's Health Initiative—one might wonder if it's ethical to deprive one-half of all women in the study of estrogen's proven life-saving benefits. Frankly, the whole thing disturbs me. If this study continues, we'll eventually have a large amount of "data"—namely the numbers of *women who died prematurely*—to consider.

Estrogen and Breast Cancer Survivors

Currently, approximately four million breast cancer survivors are living in the United States. The majority of these women are postmenopausal. But there are also substantial numbers of younger women in this group, women who have been treated with chemotherapy and have gone through menopausal changes at an earlier age.

Physicians have long been concerned that giving estrogen to women who have a history of breast cancer might be considered as "adding fuel to the fire," or that using estrogen might awaken a sleeping microscopic metastasis, and thus shorten a woman's life. Consequently, a mainstay of the prudent practice of medicine has long been that patients with breast cancer (past or present) should *not* be given estrogen.

Now, clinicians and researchers are slowly and carefully beginning to consider whether this ever-growing population of women might actually benefit, perhaps even have a survival *advantage*, with estrogen-replacement therapy.

This reappraisal is based mainly on the following facts:

- Estrogen's protective effects against heart disease and osteoporosis, its maintenance of cognitive function, and its relief of menopausal symptoms are all well established.

- The very high hormonal levels of estrogen that women experience during pregnancy have no effect on breast cancer survival. Additionally, breast cancer survivors who have had subsequent pregnancies are not adversely affected.
- The use of oral contraceptives at doses 2 to 4 times higher than that used in current estrogen-replacement therapy has no effect on breast cancer risk.
- Women who were taking estrogen-replacement therapy at the time their breast cancer was diagnosed actually *survived longer*, with a reduced mortality rate, than did women who were not taking hormones at the time of diagnosis.

Let's take a closer look at these intriguing findings.

Microscopic breast cancer is present in the body from five to eight years before a breast cancer tumor is large enough to be detected. So it is safe to assume that many pregnant women and many women on birth-control pills were inadvertently, or "accidentally," exposed to high levels of estrogen while harboring breast cancer cells. And yet careful analysis has revealed *no* effect on breast cancer survival. These clusters of breast cancer cells are apparently *not* stimulated to grow when exposed to the hormones of pregnancy or to birth-control pills.

Even more impressive are the studies involving women who were on hormone-replacement therapy before their breast cancers were diagnosed. These women were also "accidentally" taking estrogen for years because they were "on the pill" while they were harboring breast cancer cells in their body. And yet several large studies have found *improved* survival rates among women taking estrogen (compared with women not taking estrogen) at the time of their breast cancer diagnosis:

- Gambrel reported a mortality rate of 22 percent for women on estrogen-replacement therapy at the time of diagnosis of breast cancer, versus 46 percent for those not taking hormones.
- Hunt reported a 45 percent *reduction* in mortality in women who were taking estrogen at the time of diagnosis of breast cancer in a study of 4,500 women on estrogen-replacement therapy.
- Bergkvist followed 261 women for nine years who were using estrogen at the time of breast cancer diagnosis. He compared these women with a population of 6,600 women who were not taking estrogen at the time of their breast cancer diagnosis. At the end of eight years there were 40 percent *fewer* mortalities in the group who took estrogen.
- In the light of these data, Dr. Philip DiSaia, a nationally recognized expert in gynecological cancer, studied forty-one women who elected to receive estrogen-replacement therapy after diagnosis and treatment of breast cancer. They were matched to eighty-two women who did not receive estrogen. There were no differences in survival or disease progression for periods of up to eleven years.
- Brewster and DiSaia further reported on 145 breast cancer survivors who elected to receive hormone-replacement therapy. Half of the patients began therapy within three years of diagnosis and one-third of the patients delayed estrogen-replacement therapy until six years after diagnosis. The overall

recurrence rate was not increased. As stated by the authors, "Our limited experience does not suggest an adverse outcome associated with estrogen replacement."

Most practicing physicians in the United States simply do not offer estrogen-replacement therapy to their patients who are breast cancer survivors. This well-intentioned advice has been based on the fundamental tenet of the practice of medicine: *Prime non nocere*—First, do no harm. In light of the insight provided by the current studies, however, perhaps it is time to carefully re-evaluate this approach. Although we do not, as yet, have the definitive answer, it may now be appropriate, after detailed and open discussion between doctor and patient, to offer breast cancer survivors the benefits of estrogen-replacement therapy.

Concluding Thoughts

It's all about perspective. Estrogen can save too many lives to let fear of breast cancer keep women from securing its benefits.

Based on available evidence, in any group of women taking estrogen from age fifty to age seventy-five, there will be 3 percent to 6 percent more survivors at age seventy-five than in a comparable group of women *not* taking estrogen. In the next millennium, this will involve more than 30 million women in the United States. This means that estrogen has the potential to save the lives of one to two million women in the United States in the early part of the twenty-first century.

Since its message is the central thesis of this book, my analysis of breast cancer statistics was outlined in the in-

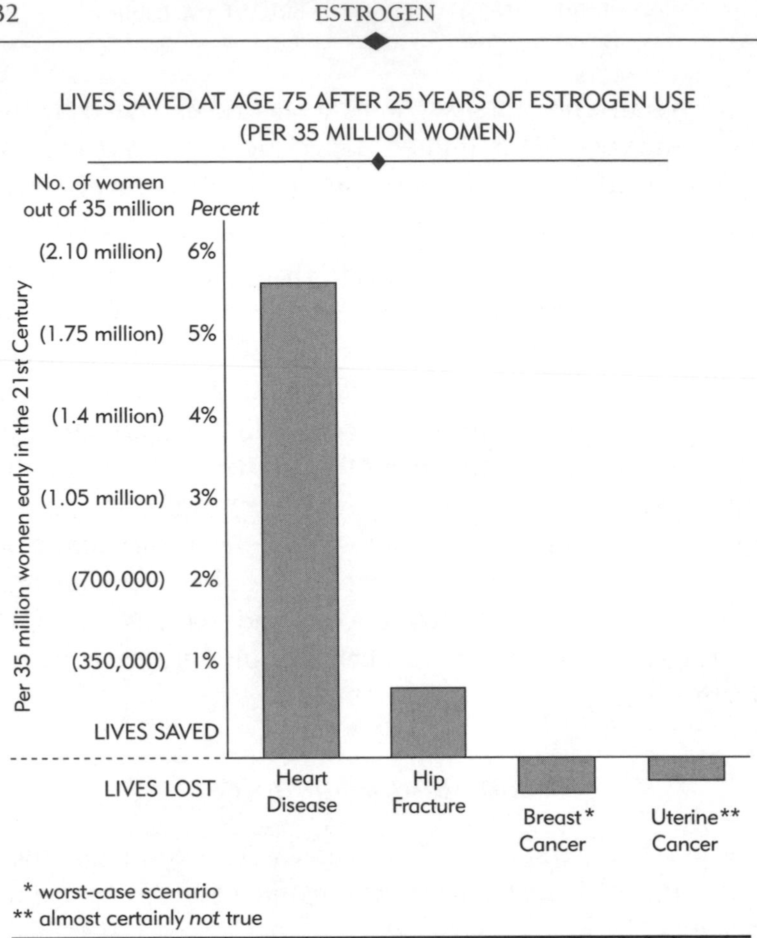

troduction. I now want to underscore it, because it is critical to how we perceive the issues surrounding breast cancer and estrogen. Here is the basis of my analysis:

> 10,000 women take estrogen from age 50 to age 75
> 10,000 women do not take estrogen
> At age 75, one study predicts approximately:

- 567 lives saved from heart disease.
- 75 lives saved from hip fracture.
- 39 lives lost to breast cancer.

This represents a total of 642 lives saved against 39 lives lost. Six hundred women's lives saved out of every group of 10,000 is a total of 6 percent. Even using a more conservative estimate regarding heart disease, which some researchers do, with estrogen use the lives of at least 3 percent of women will be prolonged.

The bottom line: Estrogen prolongs the lives of 3.5 to 6.5 percent of menopausal women. Increased breast cancer *might* possibly tug these numbers down by half a percentage point. The irony is that women's fear of this 0.5 percent risk is causing them to miss the 3 to 6 percent advantage.

In other words, about 20,000 to 60,000 preventable premature deaths will occur in the United States every year simply because the majority of women are not taking estrogen.

You can reread this chapter or peruse as much published work as you wish. The basic themes about estrogen and breast cancer will stay the same:

- Short-term use of estrogen (up to five years) does *not* increase breast cancer.
- Long-term use of estrogen *might* cause a small increase. Even though the data are weak and unconvincing, we will just have to bear this in mind until the final answer is in. (I think the answer will be that estrogen does *not* cause the loss of *any* additional lives to breast cancer—and may even *reduce* the mortality rate, as some studies have indicated.)

Hopefully—in light of the profound life-preserving benefits of estrogen on heart disease and osteoporosis, and its potentially remarkable reduction of Alzheimer's disease—estrogen use will grow, saving more lives, even in the face of a *possible* small increase in breast cancer.

Key Points to Consider*

▶ Short-term use of estrogen (up to five years) does not increase breast cancer.

▶ Long-term use of estrogen might cause a small increase. The profoundly large and proven life-preserving benefits of estrogen overwhelm estrogen's small, and as yet unproven, negative effect on breast cancer.

▶ In a recent Gallup poll, *40 percent* of women believed they were going to die from breast cancer. This is *ten times* higher than the accepted truth, which is that *4 percent* of women die from breast cancer. In fact, more than 40 percent of women will die from *cardiovascular disease,* not breast cancer. And yet only 10 percent of the women polled listed that as their primary concern.

▶ Consider that oral contraceptives contain doses of estrogen and progestin about two to four times higher than those used in hormone-replacement therapy, and yet they have no effect on breast cancer risk.

▶ The high levels of estrogen and progesterone found in pregnancy have no effect on breast cancer risk.

▶ Women who were taking estrogen-replacement therapy at the time their breast cancer was diagnosed have been shown to survive *longer,* with a reduced mortality rate, than women who were not taking hormones at the time of diagnosis.

▶ Based on available evidence, in any group of women taking estrogen from age fifty to age seventy-five, there will be

*In most chapters, I have included a "Key Points to Consider" box for quick reference to the material, which is conveyed more substantively within the chapters themselves.

3 to 6 percent more survivors at age seventy-five than in a comparable group of women not taking estrogen.

► In the next millennium, 30 million women in the United States will be age fifty to seventy-five. This means that estrogen has the potential to save the lives of one to two million women in the early part of the twenty-first century.

► Again, estrogen prolongs the lives of 3 to 6 percent of menopausal women. Increased breast cancer might possibly tug these numbers down by half a percentage point. The irony is that women's fear of this 0.5 percent risk is causing them to miss the 3 to 6 percent advantage. In other words, about 20,000 to 60,000 preventable premature deaths will occur in the United States every year simply because the majority of women are not taking estrogen.

2

SAVING LIVES:

Estrogen and Heart Disease

The impact of estrogen on the heart and the overriding importance of its use become clear when we keep in mind one fundamental truth: *Heart disease is far and away the leading cause of death among women.* Cardiovascular disease is responsible for nearly half (46 percent) of all women's deaths—about 500,000 deaths each year—250,000 of which are from coronary-artery disease.* Approximately 100,000 of these yearly cardiovascular deaths are *premature*; that is, they occur in women under the age of sixty-five. It is almost certain that estrogen can prevent *about one-third to one-half* of these deaths.

Bear in mind that a woman has a 23 percent risk of dying of heart disease. Contrast this with the much lower

*Coronary artery disease is caused by a buildup of plaque on the inner walls of the coronary arteries, which can ultimately block blood flow to the heart and cause heart attacks.

numbers for dying of other ailments, such as 4 percent for breast cancer, 2.5 percent for bone fractures, and 2 percent for cancers of the reproductive tract. So anything—smoking cessation, cholesterol lowering—*anything* that can make a dent in reducing such huge numbers of heart-disease victims will result in the saving of lives. Given estrogen's ability to prevent heart disease, the fact that the majority of women don't take it is tragic.

Compared to men, premenopausal women are protected against heart disease. In general, women experience coronary-artery disease ten years later than men do, and suffer fatal heart attacks twenty years later. The reason for this protection is, quite simply and precisely, estrogen.

The connection between heart disease and estrogen was established forty years ago, when researchers learned that women who had had their ovaries removed lost their cardiac protection and became similar to men as regards getting heart disease and having heart attacks. Clearly, something about a woman's biological makeup—most likely estrogen—was responsible for preventing and delaying heart disease. Since then, we have learned in great detail just how estrogen effects the cardiovascular system and why it is so protective.

Estrogen impacts cardiac health in several ways:

- *Cholesterol:* Taking estrogen affects the balance between "good" (HDL) cholesterol versus "bad" (LDL) cholesterol, not only raising the level of HDL and lowering the level of LDL, but also preventing LDL from being transformed into a more potent, harmful form.
- *Blood vessels:* Estrogen helps maintain the healthy function of the blood vessels, promoting dilatation

(widening) and thereby ensuring good blood flow to the heart and brain.

- *Atherosclerotic plaques:* Plaque is the substance that builds up inside a vessel, causing it to narrow. In an environment where estrogen is abundant, fewer plaques form and those that are already present are less likely to rupture. Plaque rupture can attract a blood clot, severely block a blood vessel, and cause a heart attack.

Cholesterol

There is still nothing wrong with the simple notion of "good" HDL (high density lipoprotein) cholesterol and "bad" LDL (low density lipoprotein) cholesterol. The concept has been based on the idea that LDL cholesterol stays in the blood-vessel wall and damages it, while HDL cholesterol pulls damaging LDL cholesterol out of the vessel back into the bloodstream.

LDL travels through the vessel wall and takes part in normal chemical processes before it is eventually removed from the vessel wall by HDL. However, these normal chemical processes create oxygen-derived "free radicals" which can attach themselves to the LDL, creating "oxidized LDL." This newly formed oxidized LDL is particularly attractive to scavenger cells in the blood vessels. These cells ingest this cholesterol, becoming bloated and abnormal.* Leftover cholesterol forms "lipid pools"—or fat deposits—in the vessel wall, beginning the process of atherosclerotic plaque formation.

When estrogen is present in the blood-vessel wall, less

*These cholesterol-filled cells are called foam cells.

oxidized LDL is formed. Here estrogen acts as an "antioxidant" (much like vitamin E), binding the free radicals before they have a chance to oxidize LDL. The less oxidized LDL that is present in the blood vessel walls, the fewer damaging atherosclerotic plaques will form.

Estrogen also affects cholesterol by stimulating the liver to manufacture less LDL and more HDL. This means less LDL to damage the vessels and more HDL to remove the LDL that does remain. *This high-HDL environment, which women enjoy during their premenopausal years, confers significant cardio-protection but is progressively lost during the menopausal years as estrogen is lost.*

Estrogen and the Blood Vessels

The fact that estrogen protects the heart by keeping cholesterol levels in check is only part of the story. It turns out that estrogen is actually involved in, and improves, almost all of the fundamental workings of a woman's cardiovascular system, including the blood vessels.

In order for the blood to effectively transport oxygen and other vital nutrients through the vessels to the tissues, the blood vessels must do much more than merely serve as a pipeline. They must be pliable, strong, and unencumbered by blood clots or the damaging plaques of atherosclerosis.

Pliability is the key. During times when the body presents an increased demand for oxygen to the tissues—such as with exercise or stress—the blood vessels must dilate to accommodate the increased blood flow necessary to deliver that extra oxygen where it is needed. A half-hour's jog provides a good example. Just minutes into your run, your heart starts pumping harder and faster in an effort to keep up with the extra oxygen required by your leg muscles and your heart—which is itself a muscle. If your legs don't get the extra oxygen they need, the worst that might happen is that your calf will cramp up and slow you down a bit. But if your *heart* is oxygen deprived, the result can be chest pain (angina) or worse, a heart attack or sudden death.

A similar situation occurs when the body is under stress, both physical and psychological. At such times, the heart pumps harder and faster and more blood is expelled. Simultaneously, the body secretes chemicals—acetylcholine and epinephrine—that send messages to the blood vessels to dilate. A normal blood vessel will dilate in response to these chemical messages to let more blood through. But if the blood vessel is diseased, it will actually *constrict*, which is exactly the opposite of what the body wants. The tissue wants *more* oxygen and blood flow—but it winds up getting *less*.

Estrogen promotes and maintains the vital ability of the blood vessels to dilate during exercise, under stress, or whenever the body calls for more blood. This process is called "vasodilatation." Vasodilatation depends on several interrelated steps: First, the inner lining of the blood vessels, the "endothelium," secretes a chemical called "nitric oxide." Next, nitric oxide causes the blood vessel to dilate. Estrogen directs the endothelium to manufacture and release nitric oxide.

In another important role, *estrogen helps to relax the muscle cells that surround the blood vessels, preventing them from squeezing and constricting the vessels at the wrong time.* When the constricted vessel in question is a coronary artery, the result is called "coronary spasm." The coronary arteries branch out like a tree across the surface of the heart and deliver oxygen that feeds the heart muscle. A constricted coronary artery shuts off blood flow and can, if it lasts too long, lead to a heart attack. *Maintaining the ability of the vessels to dilate under stress and preventing any action that constricts them may well be one of the fundamental mechanisms by which estrogen saves lives.*

And there is more. Not only does estrogen prevent heart disease, *estrogen helps even women who already have heart disease.* Recently, doctors learned that adding estrogen to a coronary artery that has gone into spasm can, within seconds, restore that artery to its normal diameter. This has been shown repeatedly and scientifically in the laboratory during coronary angiography, a procedure in which a catheter is placed in the coronary arteries, dye injected, and an X-ray outline of the blood vessels obtained.

In fact, some of the most compelling evidence of estrogen's protective effect on the heart, and against heart disease, comes from studies involving coronary angiography. *In all studies, survival is significantly higher among estrogen users.*

A study by Sullivan of more than 2,000 women with varying degrees of heart disease confirms this fact. Among other findings, the ten-year survival rate of women with *severe* heart disease was only 60 percent among women who did *not* use estrogen, compared to 97 percent of the estrogen users. This underscores the fact that women with established heart disease, even when that disease is severe, stand to benefit significantly from estrogen use. *In fact, as the severity of coronary artery disease increases, the survival advantage of estrogen users over nonusers increases.*

Topol studied the relationship between estrogen use and whether a patient's coronary arteries stayed open after various coronary procedures. He found that regardless of the procedure performed, the estrogen user's arteries stayed open to a significantly greater degree than did the arteries of the nonusers.

Gruchow studied 933 postmenopausal women in whom the degree of coronary blockage (occlusion) was measured and given a score. Estrogen users had lower blockage scores. The women over age sixty showed the greatest difference in scores. *As women aged, the degree of blockage worsened significantly in the nonusers, but remained stable in the estrogen users.*

Hong studied the angiograms of 90 postmenopausal women who were complaining of chest pain. They were divided into estrogen users and nonusers. The results of the angiograms showed that of the women on estrogen, only 22 percent had coronary-artery disease, compared to women who did not use estrogen, 68 percent of whom had coronary artery disease. Not using estrogen was the single most powerful risk factor of coronary-artery disease in these women.

It is clear that estrogen can prevent new coronary-artery disease from occurring and can stabilize existing disease—even if it is severe. *Indeed, the studies indicate that women with coronary-artery disease undergoing bypass surgery should be encouraged to take estrogen postoperatively to improve survival.*

Estrogen and the Biology of the Plaques

The final component for efficient blood flow to the heart is a clear, unobstructed blood vessel. Normally, the lining of a blood vessel—the endothelium—is smooth and unbroken. Any injury or break in the endothelium, even the smallest tear, can begin several processes, none of them good: plaque formation, inflammation, and clotting.

When the endothelium of a vessel is injured, as can happen, for example, when blood courses at high pressure through a vessel with no "give," nature attempts to repair the damage. Immediately, cells begin to proliferate and divide. In the course of this repair process, scavenger cells absorb excessive amounts of cholesterol (particularly the artery's nemesis, oxidized LDL cholesterol). When these scavenger cells in the blood-vessel walls fill with lipids, particularly oxidized LDL, fat deposits form. And, as we've discussed, it is precisely these fat deposits that lead to the formation of plaque. The plaque then rises up through the injured endothelium and bulges threateningly into the center of the artery.

At this point, another biological process takes place. A "fibrous cap" grows over the protrusion, acting as a barrier between the rough-edged plaque and the bloodstream. If the cap remains stable and the vessel has not been narrowed significantly, blood will continue to flow normally around the protrusion. But if a break occurs in the fibrous cap covering the plaque, inflammation and clotting can occur.

Unfortunately, a blood clot (called a "thrombus") may not always stay small. Sometimes it continues to grow until finally it becomes large enough to completely close off the blood vessel. Or sometimes just a small piece of the newly formed clot may break off, travel through the bloodstream, and lodge in a narrower vessel downstream. This type of clot is called an "embolus." In either case, if such an event occurs in one of the coronary arteries, the result may well be a heart attack or sudden death.

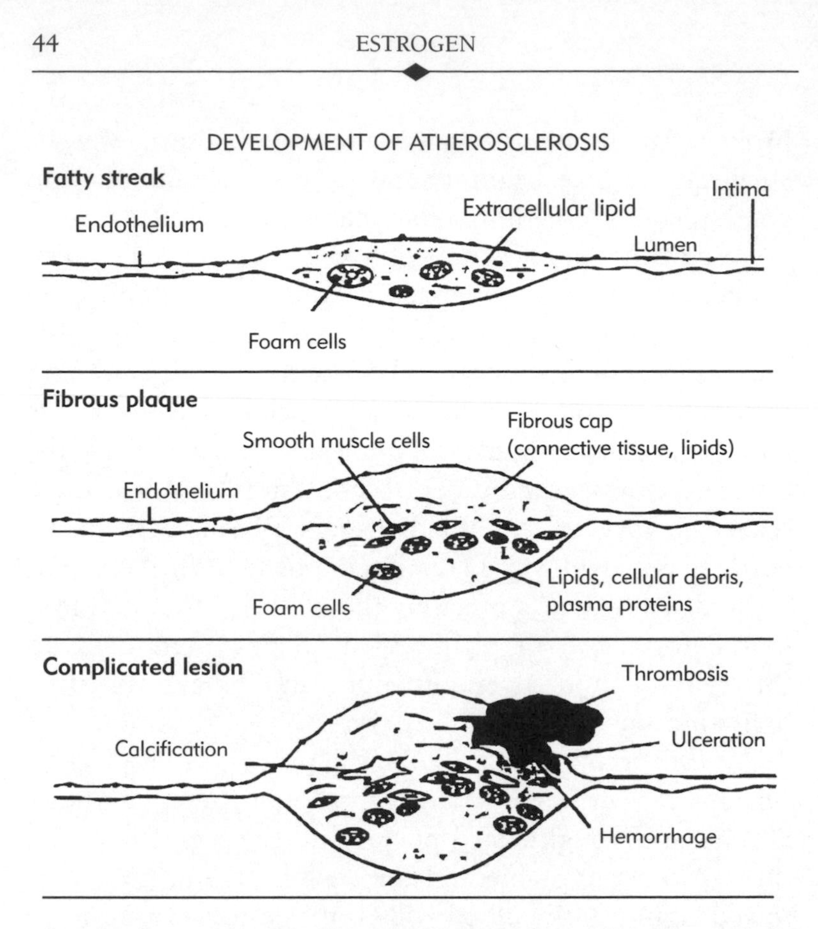

From R.L. Byyny and L. Speroff, *A Clinical Guide for Care of Older Women, 2nd ed.*, Baltimore: Williams and Wilkins, 1996.

So, quite simply, the idea is to try to prevent plaque formation, and to allow those plaques that are already formed to be stabilized so that their protective caps don't break. *Estrogen does both of these things.*

Estrogen protects the blood vessels by:

- Increasing HDL and lowering LDL, thereby shifting the balance in favor of removing cholesterol from the artery wall
- Preventing the oxidation of LDL into the far more toxic oxidized LDL, which can accelerate the process of plaque formation
- Preventing the cells of the artery wall from overgrowing in response to injury, thereby stopping the growth of plaque before it starts
- Allowing a stable fibrous cap to develop, which prevents plaque from being exposed to the turbulence of the bloodstream
- Decreasing the inflammatory response associated with injury, which, if unchecked, can weaken the fibrous cap
- Changing the level of chemicals to prevent clots from forming on the plaque
- Allowing the vessel to dilate when necessary, which facilitates the flow of increased amounts of blood over the plaque without creating excessive pressure, which could disturb the vessel wall or cause a break in the fibrous cap

Estrogen's Effects on Insulin and Diabetes

It turns out that too much insulin is bad for you. Insulin has a direct effect on blood vessels that results in increased plaque formation. Further, it increases a chemical (endothelin-I) that causes the blood vessels to constrict.

Insulin levels are lower in women taking estrogen. This results in two excellent benefits—namely, less atherosclerotic damage and constriction of blood vessels, and less incidence of diabetes. Indeed, the Nurses Health Study reported a 20 percent reduction in the incidence of diabetes among estrogen users. A quite recent study by Schultz and Lambert of approximately 400 women revealed a provocative finding: Of 36 women who developed diabetes, 31 had never used estrogen and only 5 were from the group of estrogen users. In yet another recent study by Dr. Karen Friday, even women with preexisting diabetes have lower blood sugars while on estrogen, reflecting the fact that estrogen makes it easier for insulin to lower blood sugar.

How estrogen accomplishes this is actually an interesting story. In the low-estrogen environment after menopause, women increase their abdominal fat (which used to be on the hips). This abdominal fat is not only a nuisance, it actually makes the body more resistant to insulin. To counter this "insulin resistance," the body produces *more* insulin—which is not good for the health of blood vessels.

In contrast, when estrogen is replaced, abdominal fat is reduced and any insulin resistance diminishes, or is entirely eliminated. If all goes according to plan, what results is less insulin, better cardiovascular health, fewer cases of diabetes, *and* a more favorable relationship between your waist and your hips.

What About Stroke?

Estrogen provides highly significant protection against strokes. A stroke occurs when a clot that develops somewhere else in the circulation breaks off and travels to the brain, lodging in an artery and causing damage to any brain tissue that depends on that particular artery for oxygen. Although years ago high levels of estrogen, as was found in older high-dose birth-control pills, were linked to blood clots and stroke, there is now clear evidence that at current low doses it *does not* increase the risk of stroke.

Given estrogen's beneficial effects against cardiovascular disease—maintaining healthy blood-vessel function, decreasing the number and stabilizing the structure of the plaques, and preventing clot formation—this comes as no surprise. In one study of nearly 9,000 female residents of the Leisure World Retirement Community in California, those who took estrogen had a 46 percent overall *reduction* in the risk of death from stroke. This included women with high blood pressure and those who smoked. Another study of 23,000 women in Upsala, Sweden, showed a 30 percent reduction in the occurrence of strokes in women who used estrogen-progestin combinations.

In yet another study, the National Health and Nutrition Examination Survey (NHANES) recruited nearly 2,000 postmenopausal women in the early 1970s. *Estrogen use in this group was associated with a 31 percent reduction in the occurrence of stroke and a highly significant 63 percent reduction in death from stroke.*

The Nurses Health Study, begun in 1976 and comprising 70,000 postmenopausal women, has not as yet shown a protective connection between stroke and estrogen use. However, many researchers expect that, as the population of nurses gets older and strokes begin to occur in more significant numbers, a protective effect may become apparent.

What About Blood Pressure?

Estrogen does not raise blood pressure. Period.

In fact, one study showed that estrogen actually reduced diastolic blood pressure (the pressure when the heart is at rest). In one recent study of seventy-five women in a hypertension clinic, no significant changes were found. This was confirmed by yet another study of hypertensive patients.

What About Phlebitis and Blood Clots?

Phlebitis, or venous thrombophlebitis, occurs when clots form in veins (usually in the legs) and cause inflammation. Sometimes clots that began in the leg can break off and travel to the lungs (pulmonary embolus), which can have serious consequences.

In contrast to the studies regarding stroke, the data regarding estrogen's effect on blood clots are somewhat mixed, with some recent studies showing an increased risk among estrogen users. But the majority of the studies have shown no effect. Fortunately, the incidence of phlebitis is low, about 1 in 10,000, and serious consequences are uncommon. At most, hormone-replacement therapy causes one extra case in 5,000 women. In my judgment, this is not clinically significant.

Until recently, because of the history that linked high-dose birth-control pill to blood clots, physicians have not prescribed estrogen to patients with hypertension, heart disease, or increased risk of stroke. It is these very same patients, however, who *should* be taking estrogen.

What About Progesterone?

In the past two decades, we have learned that women with their uterus intact must take progesterone along with estrogen to counteract estrogen's growth-promoting effect on uterine cells. So the question is: Does taking progesterone counteract the beneficial effects of estrogen on blood vessels and the heart? Fortunately, from the broadest perspective, the news is good. *Estrogen with progesterone added seems to save just as many lives as estrogen alone.*

There is, however, still some concern. Up to this point, we have seen that estrogen does nothing but good in terms of cholesterol, the heart, and the blood vessels. The same cannot be said about all the compounds that are often lumped together and called progesterone.*

- *Stronger* progestins are artificial compounds often found in birth-control pills. They are much stronger than natural progesterone and can produce slightly more male (androgenic) side effects.
- *Weaker* progestins are closer structurally to progesterone. *Provera* (medroxyprogesterone), which is far and away the most commonly used progestin in the United States, falls into this category.
- *Natural* progesterone is identical to a woman's own progesterone. It has only recently become available as an oral medication. Because scientists couldn't figure out a way to prevent its disintegration in the stomach, it has had to be administered vaginally.

*The compounds here are called, colloquially, progesterone. However, in medical terms, artificial progesterone compounds are referred to as progestins. Only "natural" progesterone is medically known as progesterone.

> Now that an oral form is available, its use may increase substantially.

Some of the progestins can have adverse effects: For example, some of the beneficial effects of estrogen on HDL and LDL cholesterol levels are reduced. This is especially true with the use of the stronger progestins. There is also some evidence that progestins (but not "natural" progesterone) can possibly reduce estrogen's effect on vasodilatation. And some studies show that the progestins can cause spasm of the coronary arteries—although, again, this does not seem to be true of "natural" progesterone.

With this evidence, it is logical to expect that estrogen's benefits would be reduced or even neutralized when it is combined with progestin. But in fact, this has been largely disproven. The most reassuring scientific evidence by far comes from a particular part of the Nurses Health Study of 48,000 women, which has demonstrated *absolutely no reduction* in estrogen's benefits when progestin is added. Other studies appear to confirm this.

Frankly, this is in some ways a lucky break. It probably means that estrogen does so many positive things to the cardiovascular system that it overrides any potential negative effects of progestins.

At this point, it seems to me that we should be actively examining precisely which form of progesterone to use and in what dose it should be given. Personally, I think the stronger progestins now popular in Europe should be avoided. Provera, which is weaker, seems preferable because it has fewer negative effects on cholesterol. Best of all might be "natural" progesterone, which has minimal, if any, negative effects on cholesterol and may not cause any spasm of the blood vessel. However, recent studies have not shown any difference between the effects of "natural" progesterone and Provera on cholesterol levels. Since the use of "natural" progesterone has been limited to date, we'll have to let time pass to judge its true efficacy.

Concluding Thoughts

Though the details might seem daunting, estrogen's multiple benefits to the cardiovascular system are clear. By helping prevent the formation of atherosclerotic plaques, estrogen attacks heart disease early in its course. By helping the blood vessels to open and remain open, estrogen not only allows the heart to get much-needed oxygen, it allows the plaques already formed to stabilize and thus prevents clot formation and its devastating consequences. And the idea that estrogen actually helps the diseased blood vessel dilate when under stress, thereby prolonging life even in the presence of severe coronary artery disease, is truly remarkable.

Indeed, of the more than thirty published studies on estrogen and the heart, only a handful have failed to find evidence for estrogen's protective effects. *The general consensus is that estrogen decreases the risk of heart disease by about 50 percent, representing a potential savings of tens of thousands of women's lives each year in the United States.* I hope that, in light of these newly discovered effects of estrogen on heart disease, taking estrogen will now seem much more a matter of *logic* and less a matter of faith.

Key Points to Consider

- The general consensus is that estrogen decreases the risk of heart disease by about 50 percent, representing a potential savings of tens of thousands of women's lives each year in the United States.

- Not only does estrogen prevent heart disease, estrogen helps even women who already have heart disease. In all studies of women with heart disease, survival is shown to be significantly higher among estrogen users.

- Maintaining the ability of blood vessels to dilate under stress and preventing any action that constricts them may well be one of the fundamental mechanisms by which estrogen saves lives.

- Insulin levels are lower in women taking estrogen. This results in two excellent benefits—less atherosclerotic damage and constriction of blood vessels, and less incidence of diabetes.

- Estrogen provides highly significant protection against strokes.

- Estrogen does not raise blood pressure.

3

ESTROGEN AND THE BRAIN:

Modern Wonders

Our humanity is defined by our hearts and minds. Yet the fundamental manner by which our brain provides thoughts and emotions still remains beyond our grasp, seeming more the stuff of magic than scientific endeavor. Consequently, this particular field of inquiry—the effects of estrogen on how we think and feel—must be approached with extraordinary humility.

Although acquiring new knowledge is exciting, at best we're developing only a "sense" of estrogen's effect on the structure and function of the brain. Nonetheless, keeping in mind our scant and often conflicting database, let's examine some truly fascinating findings regarding the effects of estrogen on:

- *Mood*: That estrogen improves mood has been widely accepted for some time; however, theories regarding how it does so are quite new.

- *Memory and cognition*: Estrogen has specific effects that improve some, but not all, aspects of memory (though many women perceive that with estrogen, their memories are improved overall). That estrogen improves both memory and cognition by actually causing the individual brain cells to change their anatomic structure is nothing short of miraculous. In addition, estrogen alters certain aspects of brain chemistry and enhances blood flow to the brain; both functions also work in favor of cognition and memory.
- *Alzheimer's disease*: There is increasing evidence that estrogen *delays* or actually *prevents* the onset of Alzheimer's disease. In view of the extraordinary number of women affected by this disease—40 percent of women over the age of eighty—any degree of prevention, or even delay, is highly significant.
- *Balance*: Studies show that estrogen improves balance in many women who take it. Preventing falls may be another mechanism—beyond estrogen's physical benefits to the bones—by which estrogen thwarts bone fractures.

Estrogen and Mood

Estrogen enhances mood. Because estrogen also relieves distressing physical symptoms of menopause—such as hot flashes—which in and of themselves can lead to impairment of mood, researchers have tried to determine whether estrogen improves mood in menopausal women indirectly, by alleviating physical symptoms, or directly, by performing some action on the brain.

In fact, it does both. Estrogen helps to modulate the production of serotonin in the brain. Serotonin is a neurotransmitter ("neuro" = nerves, "transmitter" = message sender) that lifts the spirits and provides an overall sense of well-being. Increasing the levels of serotonin elevates mood. When serotonin levels fall, mood levels are depressed.

Estrogen increases the level and availability of serotonin by three mechanisms:

- *Estrogen "frees up" tryptophan.* Tryptophan is a naturally occurring amino acid* that is carried by cells to the brain, where it is turned into serotonin. In order for this transformation to occur, however, tryptophan must first be released from its binding sites on the cell that transports it. Estrogen disconnects tryptophan from its binding sites.
- *Estrogen decreases the enzyme monoamine oxidase (MAO).* Serotonin is prey to MAO, which has a strong affinity for this mood-elevating chemical and consumes it at every chance. Estrogen acts as an "MAO inhibitor," harnessing MAO and thereby allowing more serotonin to travel freely in the body. A whole class of antidepressant drugs was created using this mechanism. (A newer class of antidepressants has been designed specifically to increase serotonin levels through a different mechanism. Examples of these more popular drugs are Prozac and Zoloft.)
- *Estrogen increases the ability of serotonin to travel throughout the body.* Serotonin is transported in the bloodstream on the surface of platelets. Estrogen

*Amino acids are the building blocks of protein.

> increases the serotonin "seating capacity" on the platelets, thereby allowing more serotonin to be delivered to the various tissues of the nervous system.

A number of important studies have confirmed estrogen's mood-enhancing effects. One study utilized an experimental design called a "double-blind crossover." In a "double-blind" study, neither the person taking the drug nor the researcher knows whether the medication is real or a placebo. "Crossover" means that for the first half of the study the patients take one type of pill (real or placebo), and then they "cross over" and take the alternate pill for the second half. In this manner, each group spends half the time on the real drug and the other half on the placebo.

Barbara Sherwin, Ph.D., a highly regarded researcher from McGill University in Canada who specializes in the investigation of estrogen's effects on the brain, used this method to evaluate the negative moods—the study referred to this as "depression scores"—of women undergoing simultaneous hysterectomy and oophorectomy (removal of the ovaries). The women were tested immediately after their operations. For the next three months they received either hormone treatment or placebo. After this initial period, treatment was stopped and the women retested. A month later, after blood levels in both groups returned to normal, the groups switched for another three-month trial. During *both* halves of the trial, the women using hormones had *lower* depression scores than the women taking the placebo.

In another study, Dr. Sherwin looked at two groups of women four years after they had undergone oophorectomy. Those women who had been taking estrogen or an estrogen-androgen (testosterone) combination since their surgery had more positive moods than a matched group of women who had not received treatment.

A recent European study investigated the quality of life after menopause. Five hundred women were randomized into two groups to compare the way mood is affected by two different drugs: Veralipride, a drug widely used in Europe to relieve hot flashes, and estrogen. The women were asked to answer a questionnaire which incorporated five sources: The Global Women's Health Questionnaire, The Psychological General Well-Being Index, a sleep-problem questionnaire, a sexual-behavior questionnaire, and a questionnaire examining social aspects of life. The women who used hormones answered "good" or "very good" to questions about the quality of thier lives in 91 percent of cases. In contrast, with just the relief of hot flashes provided by Veralipride, only 50 percent reported they felt "good" to "very good" in terms of general well-being.

Not all past scientific research linking mood and estrogen has been as consistently positive as the above examples. In some cases, different tests, drug regimens, and research methods have yielded conflicting results. But for the most part, accumulated scientific evidence, especially when viewed from the perspective of modern concepts and theory, provides strong support for estrogen's overall beneficial effect on mood.

It should be noted that while studies show that estrogen in conventional doses enhances mood in women who are not depressed, these doses do *not* effect women who are clinically depressed. To treat clinical depression with estrogen would require doses of estrogen far too high to be considered safe.

The Effect of Estrogen on Memory and Cognition

In one of Dr. Sherwin's articles, she quoted a study on cognition: For one year, twenty-eight elderly women were given weekly injections of either estrogen or a placebo. At the end of the year, verbal IQ scores had *increased* in the women given estrogen and *decreased* in those receiving the placebo. In addition, the women who took estrogen had *improved* memory scores, while those who didn't take it showed a *decrease* in memory. A year after therapy was stopped, the scores returned to pretreatment levels, clearly indicating that improvement of memory and IQ occurred *only while estrogen was being taken.*

The notion that you can enlist a seventy-five-year-old woman who has never taken estrogen, offer her estrogen, and have her reap the benefits is truly astonishing. Even more surprising was to learn that this study, which foreshadowed all that is new and exciting about the effects of estrogen on memory and cognition, was done in 1952. (I was *born* in 1952!)

A later, equally important study tested a group of seventy-five-year-old women using the Hospital Adjustment Scale to measure the variables of communication, interpersonal relationships, ability to administer self-care, and work activities. The scores of estrogen-treated women *improved steadily* in all categories for eighteen months, then remained stable at this high point. The scores of those who were treated with a placebo *decreased steadily*, which is to be expected, given the ages of the women and the fact that with time, normal biology reduces the number of healthy cells in the body.

By the end of the 1970s, a number of studies had provided strong evidence that estrogen improves and/or maintains verbal abilities and verbal memory, as well as improving aspects of social and physical functioning in elderly women. But this was also close to the period when estrogen was being linked to uterine cancer. As a result, prevailing medical opinion was overridden by fear, and enthusiasm for estrogen waned.

Today, with current long-term estrogen use hovering at about 20 percent of women, it seems we have to discover estrogen all over again. This time around, however, we are armed with far more detailed and relevant information.

Witness, for example, the following extraordinary concepts regarding estrogen's effect on the brain and memory:

• *Estrogen can change the size and structure of brain cells.* The surface of every cell in the brain gives rise to a forest of small, tree-like structures called dendrites. These dendrites branch out into even smaller offshoots known as dendritic spines. Brain cells communicate by reaching out to each other with their dendritic spines. The greater the number of dendrites and dendritic spines on each cell, the greater the capability for interaction between them. And the greater the interaction, the better the brain can process information. This is particularly true in the hippocampus, the area of the brain responsible for decision-making, learning, and memory.

With age—and not necessarily old age—comes a natural loss of dendrites and dendritic spines and, subsequently, a loss of some memory. So any way these structures can be preserved and protected can make a vast difference in our recall. In wondrous fashion, estrogen helps preserve and protect a cell's dendrites and dendritic spines. Better still, estrogen can *increase* the number of dendritic spines on the brain cell—*within seventy-two hours* of the cell's exposure to estrogen.

It turns out that the brain is far more changeable than ever before imagined. In 1990, Dr. Bruce McEwen, a renowned scientist at Rockefeller University in New York City, showed that the adult brain is neither static nor limited to inevitable deterioration. Rather, he showed, it has *plasticity*, which means it can be chemically and structurally remodeled.

McEwen's research demonstrated through experiments on animals that when estrogen levels drop, the density of dendrites declines. He also proved that estrogen at normally high levels maintains the structural integrity of the nerve cells and, as noted above, can even increase the number of dendritic spines.

- *Estrogen participates in the manufacture of acetylcholine, which directly affects memory.* Acetylcholine is a neurotransmitter, like serotonin. But while serotonin is involved with mood changes, acetylcholine is important to memory function. Normally, acetylcholine declines as we age, contributing to our diminishing ability to remember. Estrogen helps keep memory levels elevated by increasing the manufacture of an enzyme that helps produce acetylcholine. The object is to have as much acetylcholine in the central nervous system as possible. Acetylcholine-based nerve function, especially as it pertains to memory, is significantly lacking in patients with Alzheimer's disease.

These revolutionary findings provide a rationale for using past research (the effects of estrogen on memory and cognition) as a starting point for areas of future research (the prevention and treatment of Alzheimer's disease). There is, however, another rather quaint notion linking the past to the future, namely that the brains of men and women develop differently. I shall now dare to describe this.

It begins in the womb. The hormonal environment—that is, the relative amounts of "male" testosterone and "female" estrogen—affects the development of the brain in the growing fetus. Under different hormonal influences, some neural pathways become better developed than others. Under the influence of estrogen, women tend to excel in verbal abilities, perceptual speed, memory, and fine motor skills. Due to increased testosterone, men excel in spatial and quantitative abilities and gross motor strength. Although men have a somewhat increased incidence of learning disabilities, there is no difference between the sexes in overall IQ.

In sum, since the brains of women develop under the influence of estrogen, they will have nerve cells and pathways of nerve cells which *depend* on estrogen and are *maintained* by estrogen—more so than men. Consequently, the maintenance of these pathways in women may not only improve their memory and cognition, but may delay or prevent Alzheimer's disease.

Estrogen and Alzheimer's Disease

Alzheimer's disease is primarily an age-related disease that preferentially affects 4.5 million American women and claims more than 100,000 lives annually. Women get Alzheimer's disease more than men at a ratio that ranges from 2 to 1 to 3 to 1. One theory for the higher incidence in women is that women live longer than men, which increases their chances. Another theory professes that men don't get Alzheimer's disease as often because despite aging, men continue to produce testosterone, some of which will be converted to estrogen.

Approximately 40 percent of women over the age of eighty are affected by Alzheimer's disease. As the numbers continue to climb, scientists are rushing to find a treatment that prevents, delays, or ameliorates this frightening ailment. Current thinking is that estrogen therapy may well be one of the answers.

Several recent studies have been designed to assess the effectiveness of estrogen in healthy women as well as in women who already have Alzheimer's disease. Results are showing that estrogen can be helpful in both the prevention and treatment of Alzheimer's disease in postmenopausal women.

Estrogen's Impact on the Delay and Prevention of Alzheimer's Disease

Alzheimer's disease is characterized by a buildup of protein deposits called B-amyloid, which is detrimental to brain tissue. In an effort to clear away this unwanted protein and to rid the area of any injured or dead nerve cells, the body activates helper cells, called glia. Sometimes, though, these glia cells become overzealous and emit an excessive amount of the powerful chemicals that were supposed to be helpful in the cleanup process. One such chemical, IL-I, tends to inflame and damage the nerve cells. (Inflamed nerve cells are a hallmark of Alzheimer's disease.) A second chemical, S-100b, actually stimulates the production of B-amyloid protein. And since B-amyloid is the protein that created the trouble in the first place, the process becomes an unrelenting cycle.

Estrogen breaks this cycle. The interplay between estrogen and Alzheimer's disease is as follows:

- Alzheimer's disease decreases acetylcholine—a neurotransmitter important to memory—which adversely affects the neural pathways that respond to acetylcholine. *Estrogen increases the manufacture of acetylcholine.*
- *Estrogen induces the glia cells to produce fewer inflammation-causing chemicals* (IL-I), and fewer chemicals that cause increased production of the amyloid protein that starts the disease process (S-100b).
- *Estrogen acts as an antioxidant.* Part of the toxic effects of inflammation on nerve cells may result from free radicals and "oxidative stress," which estrogen reduces by acting as an antioxidant.
- *Estrogen decreases the level of apolipoprotein B.* Women with an increased genetic risk of Alzheimer's disease produce increased amounts of a chemical (apolipoprotein B) which, at high levels, can increase the effect of the harmful amyloid protein.
- *Estrogen increases blood flow in the carotid arteries in the neck and ultimately brings more blood to the brain.* One study showed up to a 30 percent increase. Increased blood to the brain fosters the continuing health of brain neurons and helps the brain utilize glucose for energy. It has also been associated with lowering the risk of stroke and mini-stroke.

Many new and important studies have been published in the past five years that demonstrate estrogen's role in delaying and even preventing the onset of Alzheimer's disease in postmenopausal women. Unlike older studies, which often had to rely on women's recollections, these recent studies were done prospectively—that is, the research teams collected information on the participants *before* the presumptive onset of symptoms.

One study, directed by Richard Mayeux of Columbia University in New York, enrolled a group of 1,124 older women, all of whom were free of any symptoms related to Alzheimer's disease. Some of the women had taken or were currently taking estrogen and others had never taken it. The women were followed for a period of from one to five years. During this time, 167 of the women were eventually diagnosed with Alzheimer's disease. The study showed that *the risk of getting Alzheimer's disease in those who had used estrogen was 60 percent less than among those women who had never taken estrogen.* It also showed that those women who took estrogen longer than one year had a greater reduction in risk than those who took it for less than a year. Furthermore, the women on estrogen who eventually developed Alzheimer's disease did so significantly later in their lives than those women who had never used estrogen.

In a study done by Claudia Kawas called the Baltimore Longitudinal Study of Aging, 472 older women were followed for a period of up to sixteen years. Thirty-four women developed Alzheimer's disease. The study showed that *the risk of getting Alzheimer's disease among women who had used estrogen at any time in their lives was 50 percent lower than in women who had never used hormone-replacement therapy.*

The largest study to evaluate the effects of estrogen-replacement therapy on risk of Alzheimer's disease utilized data received directly from 8,877 women, all residents of Leisure World Laguna Hills, a retirement community in Southern California. Over the fourteen-year period, 248 women were given the diagnosis likely to represent Alzheimer's disease. Each of these women was matched by year of birth and death against five women who died and did not have Alzheimer's disease. Results showed that *the risk of developing Alzheimer's disease was 35 percent less in the estrogen users compared to the nonusers*. The risk decreased significantly as the dosages and duration of therapy increased. In other words, *the longer the women were on estrogen and the higher the dose, the less likely were their chances of developing Alzheimer's disease.*

Estrogen as a Treatment for Alzheimer's Disease

To date, a number of research studies have evaluated estrogen's efficacy in treating women with Alzheimer's disease. The studies have looked at variables ranging from memory, attention span, and social integration to the performance of day-to-day activities. Although the number of women enrolled in each study was small and the duration short, the results have been striking.

The women with Alzheimer's disease who were treated with estrogen scored higher on most tests of psychosocial skills than did those who received a placebo or simply did not take estrogen. The studies also showed that women less severely affected did better than those more severely effected; that higher doses seemed to afford even greater protection; and that in all areas, the effects lasted only so long as treatment continued. As with other areas of the body, for the brain to maintain estrogen's benefits, long-term use is key.

In view of recent and past research and the provocative modern theories, it appears that estrogen has remarkable benefits regarding the prevention, stabilization, and possible improvement of Alzheimer's disease. In sum, *modern studies demonstrate a 30 to 60 percent reduction in occurrence of Alzheimer's disease in estrogen users, along with significant cognitive improvements in those women already affected.*

Estrogen Improves Balance

The incidence of "wrist"* fractures increases dramatically in the first five years after menopause. Because this is too soon to be accounted for by bone loss resulting from osteoporosis, which comes on gradually, there is a good possibility it is connected to an impairment in balance.

We all stand, walk, and in general keep our balance without ever giving a second thought as to why or how. The reason we can do these things unconsciously depends on the integrity of a combination of body parts working in concert: the inner ear, the eyes, and sensory stimuli from the muscles, tendons, skin, and joints. The input from these areas is processed in parts of the brain known as the cerebellum and brain stem. Because in women both the cerebellum and brain stem contain a great number of estrogen receptors, a loss of estrogen may induce changes in the balance system.

A study by Naessen and coworkers of postmenopausal

*This actually occurs where the forearm meets the wrist.

women showed better balance function among long-term estrogen users than among nonusers. In the study, estrogen users and estrogen nonusers were asked to stand on various flat surfaces and close their eyes. Under normal conditions, most people who stand with their eyes closed will *sway* a little back and forth. The amount and speed of this motion—the "sway velocity"—was measured in these women under a variety of experimental circumstances. The results showed that estrogen users had a significant decrease in sway velocity and therefore better balance. This finding led to the conclusion that balance function is better preserved in long-term estrogen users than in nonusers.

Balance is also fostered by a significant increase in blood flow to the cerebrum and cerebellum, which is facilitated by estrogen. Both of these factors are tremendously important, especially to older women. In a later chapter we will see the results of osteoporotic bone deterioration and its link to bone fractures. Good balance is one more way to protect against such damaging falls.

What About Progesterone and the Brain?

Few definitive studies exist that explain precisely how progesterone affects the brain. While researchers continue to investigate the connection, the most recent theories show the following: Whereas estrogen stimulates brain mechanisms, progestins may counteract this effect, although progesterone added to estrogen does not affect balance. Whereas estrogen acts as an MAO inhibitor, thereby raising serotonin levels, progesterone increases MAO somewhat, and therefore might decrease serotonin levels, leading to an impairment of mood.

The key words here are "may" and "might." In fact, no one really knows for sure which of the progestins plays a role and, more important, just how much of a role they play. Some studies have been unable to show any effect from progesterone on mood or cognition, and many patients are not affected adversely at all.

In the face of uncertainty, the best answer is for you to maintain close communication with your physician. It is helpful if both patient and doctor are willing to experiment and search for the appropriate dose and choice of progestin.

Concluding Thoughts

Over the years, remarkable discoveries have revealed how estrogen interacts with the human brain. Estrogen affects the plasticity of the brain, changing the brain's anatomy in ways that improve verbal ability and memory. Estrogen's direct effects on brain chemistry lead to enhanced mood and improve the ability of aged women to care for themselves. By improving balance, estrogen most likely inhibits falls, providing yet another mechanism by which estrogen prevents fractures.

But perhaps the most important news is that the devastating consequences of Alzheimer's disease can be significantly reduced by the use of estrogen—which may impede the development of the disease by supporting the growth, survival, and repair of nerve cells, and by protecting them from the ravages of protein deposits and inflammation. This benefit alone—estrogen's effects on Alzheimer's disease—represents the potential to improve and save the lives of millions of women.

KEY POINTS TO CONSIDER

- Estrogen improves intellectual function by altering brain chemistry and by actually changing the anatomy of the brain cells.

- Estrogen has specific effects that improve some, but not all, aspects of memory.

- That estrogen improves mood has been widely accepted for some time; however, theories regarding how it does so are quite new.

- Alzheimer's disease is primarily an age-related disease that preferentially affects 4.5 million American women and claims more than 100,000 lives annually. Approximately 40 percent of women over the age of eighty are affected by Alzheimer's disease. There is increasing evidence that estrogen delays or actually prevents the onset of Alzheimer's disease.

- Some modern studies demonstrate a 30 to 60 percent reduction in the occurrence of Alzheimer's disease in estrogen users. Estrogen may also improve cognitive function in those women already affected.

- By its beneficial effect on Alzheimer's disease, estrogen stands to improve and extend the lives of millions of women.

- Studies show that estrogen improves balance in many women who take it. Preventing falls is another mechanism—beyond estrogen's physical benefits to the bones—by which estrogen may reduce bone fractures.

4

ESTROGEN PREVENTS BONE LOSS

Fifteen to twenty percent of postmenopausal women who fracture their hip are dead within six months. Fifty percent of the survivors never return to normal life. These facts are a lot worse than many patients realize. They are a lot worse than many doctors realize. Hip fractures take lives. *Estrogen saves lives and prolongs the quality of life by reducing the number of hip fractures by one-half.*

When women lose estrogen, the architectural structure of their bones begins to weaken and becomes more susceptible to fracture. This weakened condition of bone is called *osteoporosis* (osteo = bone, porous = having pores or holes).

The Magnitude of the Problem

Osteoporosis is the twelfth leading cause of death among women today. In fact, it causes the deaths of more women than ovarian cancer, cervical cancer, and uterine cancer combined. The annual statistics associated with this disease are staggering. For example:

- 40,000 women die each year in the United States from hip fracture complications.
- 60,000 women are admitted to nursing homes each year in the United States due to complications from bone fractures.
- 250,000 hip fractures occur each year.
- 250,000 wrist/forearm fractures occur each year.
- 500,000 vertebral (spinal compression) fractures occur each year.

Here are more sobering numbers:

- It is estimated that between 25 million and 30 million women in the United States have lost enough bone mass to place them at at least *double* the risk of fracture.
- More than 50 percent of women over the age of sixty-five have vertebral fractures.
- Your lifetime risk of suffering a hip fracture is about 20 percent.

The personal toll the disease takes is even greater than the numbers indicate. Severe hip fractures lead to confinement to bed, which can lead to blood clots, stroke, and pneumonia. Vertebral fractures can cause loss of height (untreated postmenopausal women lose an average of 2.5 inches in height), chronic back pain, and deformity. This is in addition to the various pulmonary, gastrointestinal, and genitourinary problems that can result from vertebral fractures.

We know from demographic studies that osteoporosis strikes women with a family history of the disease, thin women, more white women than black women, smokers, excessive drinkers, and women with a deficiency in vitamin D and calcium. The primary risk factor, however, is the decrease in estrogen levels that occurs with natural or surgical menopause. *This effects virtually every woman* after the mean age of fifty-one (or earlier, in women who have undergone surgical removal of their ovaries).

The Ever-Changing Structure and Density of Bone

The structure and anatomy of our skeleton is dynamic and ever-changing. In fact, bone is constantly and normally being remodeled. Old bone is removed ("resorbed"), leaving something of an excavation site, and new bone fills in this gap. This ongoing process keeps the bones young and strong—it is estimated that *most of our bone is no more than eight years old.* Moreover, this process adds areas of increased strength to bone if there is an increase in physical activity. Nature's genius is beautifully evident, creating a process that can sculpt our bones to meet our changing needs.

The cells that remove old bone are called "osteoclasts." The cells that form new bone are called "osteoblasts." When all goes well, there is a balance between bone removal and replacement. Also, the two activities are "coupled"—once the excavation site is dug out (by the osteoclasts), the repair crew (osteoblasts) shows up on time.

These mechanisms do not continue to work well in the absence of estrogen. In an estrogen-poor environment, the balance shifts in favor of bone removal and resorption, and against new bone formation. Further, the two processes become "uncoupled," so that excavation sites remain unfilled for longer periods of time. This pathological process weakens the bone, leaving microscopic holes and making the bone less dense and more porous.

Bone strength is extremely sensitive to any change in its density. In fact, the strength of bone—that is, its ability to withstand the physical stresses placed on it without fracturing—is proportional to its density *squared,* or multiplied by itself. This means that if any bone deteriorates to *one-half* its former density, it is left with only *one-quarter* of its original strength ($1/2 \times 1/2 = 1/4$). You can imagine how susceptible to fracture such bone would be.

Of great clinical concern is that, in the first fifteen years after menopause, women can lose 30 percent of density from the strong "cortical" bone in the hip and long bones (arms and legs), and 50 percent of density from the honeycomb-like "trabecular" bone, which fills the vertebral bones of the spine.

To assess the strength of bone and its resistance to fracture, physicians measure *bone mineral density.* If the bone mineral density is below a certain level, a diagnosis of osteoporosis of varying degrees is made. The definitions are mathematical and related to statistical methods that many of us do our best to forget once we graduate from medical school. Nonetheless, since more than a few million women this year will sit across from their physicians and hear this diagnosis, it is important to shed some light on this issue.

The Medical Definition of Osteoporosis

When doctors test for osteoporosis, the bone density of the patient, no matter how old she is, is compared with the average bone density of young premenopausal women. However, they do "mark on a curve." To pass, all you need is a grade that is above the bottom 16 percent. (If you come in eighty-third out of one hundred, you're still okay.) To completely "flunk" and get a diagnosis of osteoporosis, your bone density has to be below the *third* percentile, which means that 97 out of 100 premenopausal women have more bone than you do.

If you score anywhere between the third and the sixteenth percentile, you are considered to have "mild" or "borderline" osteoporosis, which is called "osteopenia." Frankly, I believe the nomenclature needs rethinking. There is nothing "mild" or "borderline" about being between the third and sixteenth percentiles, which *doubles* the risk of fracture.

The diagnosis of osteoporosis is reserved for those whose bone density places them in the bottom 3 percent, where the risk of fracture is at least *quadrupled*. Even with these strict definitions, one estimate places *9 million* women in the United States today with osteoporosis. Another *17 million* women have osteopenia. Thus, at least *25 to 30 million* women are at increased risk of fracture in the United States today.

A Word About the DEXA Scan

The most sensitive and accurate scan to detect osteoporosis involves two sources of X-ray and is called the Dual X-ray Absorption, or DEXA, scan. Reflecting the cleverness of this computerized testing, the report contains detailed pictures and mathematical analysis of a woman's bone density—complete with the equivalent of percentile scores.

One interesting fact is that, in one study, *60 percent* of the women who took the test elected hormone-replacement therapy, versus only *20 percent* of the women who did not take the test. Perhaps it is an enlightening experience.

Alternative X-ray and ultrasound testing are under development, but for now, I'd hold out for the better DEXA test, even if it *is* more expensive. (Don't even get me started about the evils of managed care.) It should also be noted that most women who begin hormone-replacement therapy in timely fashion may not need routine scans.

Calcium and Bone

Any citizen of late-twentieth-century America is familiar with the importance of calcium, which, if I am not mistaken, "fortifies" virtually every foodstuff imaginable. Actually, this may not be such a bad idea, since it appears we have less calcium in our bodies now than we did years ago. One study showed that the bones of skeletons recently resurrected after two hundred years had more calcium than the average American today. This may reflect an earlier diet that was richer in calcium, and perhaps it shows that people were more physically active then.

Calcium is an essential part of bone. The body is quite resourceful when it comes to maintaining normal levels of calcium in the blood. If the body senses that blood calcium levels are low, it will compensate by:

- increasing parathyroid hormone, which stimulates osteoclasts to excavate bone to "free up" needed calcium. This process allows calcium to leave the bone and enter the circulation to better take part in vital bodily functions.

- increasing the "active" form of vitamin D—called "calcitriol" or "D_3," which is especially effective in stimulating the intestine to absorb more of the needed calcium.
- increasing various chemicals to help speed the process of bone excavation.

Although the various methods the body uses to increase blood levels of calcium can be benign, they can also be harmful if unchecked. For example, the chemicals that accelerate bone excavation can become inflammatory and perform at excessive levels, recruiting scavenger cells and stimulating the immune system. The result can be a weakening—or even increased breakdown—of bone. Estrogen alters these complex biological mechanisms at several levels.

Estrogen and the Biology of Osteoporosis

When estrogen levels decrease, the undesirable aspects of bone remodeling increase, leading to distortion of the bone architecture. Estrogen restores the balance between bone excavation by osteoclasts and bone formation by osteoblasts. In fact, estrogen interacts with bone on many levels.

For example:

- There are estrogen receptors on the bone-forming osteoblasts, which increase their activity in response to estrogen.

- Estrogen "recouples" the activity of the osteoblast to the osteoclast so that all excavation sites are filled in promptly.
- Estrogen suppresses osteoclastic activity so that there are fewer excavation sites.
- Estrogen increases the amount of highly active vitamin D_3, which stimulates the intestine to absorb more calcium.
- Estrogen increases the vitamin D receptors on osteoblasts—encouraging and increasing their bone-forming response to vitamin D.
- When the body attempts to increase calcium by secreting parathyroid hormone to "free up" calcium from bone, estrogen tempers the bone's reaction so that fewer excavation sites are created.
- Estrogen controls the amount and activity of inflammatory chemicals that can have harmful effects if unchecked.
- Estrogen stimulates the production of calcitonin, a hormone that protects bone from breaking down by decreasing the activity and number of osteoclasts.
- Estrogen stimulates the growth of collagen, a binding material found in all of the body's connective tissue that may also assist in making bone stronger.
- Through its beneficial effect on brain tissue and circulation, estrogen improves balance and may prevent falls that cause fractures.
- Through its beneficial effect on the cardiovascular system, estrogen improves exercise tolerance and performance.

But for all the good it can do, estrogen cannot halt all the effects of aging. Aging itself can result in decreased vitamin D manufactured by the kidneys, decreased calcium absorption by the intestine, and changes in bone density due to physical inactivity and decreased dietary calcium.

Nonetheless, about *75 percent* of all bone loss is due to estrogen deficiency. Estrogen will decrease hip fractures by *50 percent* and, along with calcium and vitamin D supplementation, may decrease vertebral fractures by up to *80 percent.*

Estrogen as Preventative Treatment for Osteoporosis

A large number of studies emphasize estrogen's important role in maintaining a strong bone structure and preventing osteoporosis. One representative trial, called the PEPI (Postmenopausal Estrogen/Progestin Interventions) Trial, was conducted at seven clinical centers and included 875 healthy women aged forty-five to sixty-four. The purpose was to assess the short-term health effects of four different hormone-replacement regimens: Premarin alone; Premarin with Provera added for two weeks a month; the two hormones taken together continuously; and Premarin given in sequence with micronized ("natural") progesterone.

Results of the study showed that over a period of three years, participants who took a look-alike placebo *lost* on average of 2.8 percent of spinal bone density and 2.2 percent of the hip bone density, while those who stayed on hormone therapy *gained* an average of 5.1 percent spinal bone density and 2.3 percent hip bone density. The choice of regimens made no difference. The study also showed that *hormone-replacement therapy can do more than just slow the loss of bone after menopause; it can actually increase bone mass, even in women who start using it in their sixties.*

Multiple studies have demonstrated that a standard dose of 0.625 mg of conjugated estrogen is necessary to preserve bone density. The equivalent doses of transdermal estrogen (the patch) are equally effective. The addition of a progestin has *no* negative effect and is likely to have an additional positive benefit. Similarly, in osteoporosis, the addition of testosterone is not harmful and some studies reveal a greater increase in bone density when testosterone is added.

As long as the minimal dose level of 0.625 mg of conjugated estrogen or its equivalent is maintained, the choice of any particular combination of hormones has not been found to be vitally important as regards osteoporosis.

What *is* vitally important is how long a woman stays on it. For estrogen-replacement therapy to be maximally effective in preventing fractures, it has to be taken *lifelong*. Once estrogen therapy is stopped, the result is not unlike the stroke of midnight in a children's tale: Nearly all the benefit is lost in a relatively short time. A study by Felson revealed that even if they had used estrogen for up to ten years in the past, women over seventy-five who had stopped using estrogen had only 3 percent more bone density than those who had never used estrogen at all.

In another recent study, Robert Lindsay, M.D., showed a 90 percent decrease in spinal deformities (loss of height) among surgically menopausal women who took estrogen for ten years. In his study, only 4 percent of women taking estrogen suffered spinal vertebral fractures, compared to 38 percent of untreated women.

On another positive note, reduced fractures have been reported for patients who started estrogen *after* the age of sixty-five. *Thus, it's probably never too late to start.*

The Importance of Calcium and Vitamin D as Part of Preventative Treatment

Adequate calcium intake and vitamin D are also essential for an optimal response to estrogen-replacement therapy. Women on estrogen need about 1,000 mg of calcium per day (women not taking estrogen require 1,500 mg). Since the average diet contains only 500 mg of calcium, calcium supplementation is necessary to provide the additional 500 mg for women on hormone replacement. Women over age seventy should also take 800 units of vitamin D daily. Women under age seventy who are not getting enough sunlight should take 400 to 800 units of vitamin D daily.

The Need for Estrogen as Preventative Treatment Can Occur Well Before Menopause

Although this program of prevention has focused on the elderly, the risk of developing osteoporosis is also related to the height of "peak" bone density, which is reached, surprisingly, between the ages of eighteen and thirty. Any young woman suffering from estrogen deficiency (due to anorexia, excessive physical activity, or stress-induced lack of periods) may only reach a much lower peak bone density—and therefore develop an increased risk of fracture. So clearly, women at *any* age should be vigilant about avoiding any episodes of prolonged estrogen deficiency.

Unlike many other issues surrounding hormone-replacement therapy, there is little controversy regarding the beneficial effects of estrogen on osteoporosis and fracture prevention, although estimates of the degree of these vary somewhat.

Unfortunately, 10 to 20 percent of women demonstrate "high turnover" of bone, and for these individuals standard estrogen-replacement therapy may not be maximally effective. It is possible that, with the future use of urine and blood tests, we will be able to identify these women so that individualized therapy may be initiated. When bone is broken down or formed, various specific chemicals are released in blood and urine, which can be measured—providing a "window" that enables physicians to evaluate the relative degrees of bone formation and destruction. This represents a very exciting frontier.

Concluding Thoughts

Osteoporosis is pervasive and far more deadly than we imagine, taking the lives of 40,000 women in the United States annually. Of the women who survive hip fracture, half lose degrees of independent function—many requiring surgery, hospitalization, and nursing-home care. Women with vertebral fractures lose height, which is often accompanied by spinal deformity and chronic pain. *Fifty percent* of women over the age of sixty-five have vertebral fractures.

This tremendous threat to the well-being and quality of life of postmenopausal women is being tragically undertreated, with only about 20 percent of women availing themselves of long-term estrogen treatment. Because of this, several thousand of the 40,000 lives lost each year to hip fracture are *not* prevented when they might be.

As our health care advances, the elderly population is expanding dramatically. In 1980, about 10 percent of the population was over sixty-five. This increased to 12 percent in 1990. Looking ahead to the next millennium, in 2025 nearly one in five people will be older than sixty-five. It is precisely this growing population that demands our critical thinking now. We must devote our attention and our resources to preserving the quality and length of life. Increased use of estrogen stands to have a profoundly positive effect by preventing the greater part of osteoporosis.

Key Points to Consider

► Osteoporosis is the leading cause of death among women today—40,000 women die each year in the United States from hip fracture complications alone.

► Estrogen saves lives and prolongs the quality of life by reducing the number of hip fractures by one-half.

► A woman's lifetime risk of suffering hip fracture is about 20 percent. More than 50 percent of women over the age of sixty-five have vertebral fractures.

► One estimate places *9 million* women in the United States today with osteoporosis. Another *17 million* women have osteopenia. At least *25 million to 30 million* women have lost enough bone mass to place them at at least *double* the risk of fracture.

► About *75 percent* of all bone loss is due to estrogen deficiency. As stated, estrogen will decrease hip fractures by *50 percent* and, along with calcium and vitamin D supplementation, may decrease vertebral fractures by up to *80 percent.*

► A study shows that hormone replacement therapy can do more than just slow the loss of bone after menopause; it can actually increase bone mass, even in women who start using it in their sixties.

► For estrogen-replacement therapy to be maximally effective in preventing fractures, it should be taken *lifelong.*

5

HORMONE REPLACEMENT DOES NOT CAUSE UTERINE CANCER

The storm has passed. Estrogen use *with* progesterone added almost certainly does *not* increase the incidence of uterine cancer. In fact, there is strong scientific data to support the notion that women on estrogen *and* progesterone will actually develop *fewer* cases of uterine cancer than women who don't take hormones at all. Some residual elements of controversy remain, but the data that show a small increased risk are based on statistical techniques that are much more prone to error.

In the most complete and scholarly review of nearly forty studies, Grady and colleagues tabulated the various conflicting studies on use of estrogen with progesterone added and found a 20 percent *reduction* (relative risk = 0.8)* in uterine cancer. Interestingly,

*For a more complete discussion of relative risk, refer to Appendix B.

the studies using the scientifically preferred *prospective* approach (give half the women estrogen with progesterone, give the other half a placebo, and see what happens over time) revealed a *60 percent decrease* in uterine cancer with the use of estrogen-progesterone. In my personal judgment, this is far and away the most reliable and credible finding. The less reliable *retrospective* approach (select patients with and without uterine cancer, and ask them if they ever used estrogen and progesterone) showed an increased risk (relative risk = 1.8), but the data are not nearly as powerful.

The currently accepted professional clinical opinion is that estrogen with progesterone does *not* increase the incidence of uterine cancer. Personally, I believe it most probably decreases it. The "problem" with estrogen and uterine cancer dates back to the original use of estrogen *without* the addition of protective progesterone, a treatment known as "unopposed estrogen."

Lessons from History: How Not *to Use Estrogen*

In the 1960s, doctors prescribed estrogen for menopausal women without adding progesterone. In good faith, it was presumed that one week a month off estrogen would allow the uterine lining to shed and prevent any buildup of tissue. It didn't work out that way.

In the early 1970s, it became apparent that uterine cancer was clearly increased by the use of unopposed estrogen. The longer estrogen *unopposed* by progesterone was used, the higher the risk. For example:

- Use of unopposed estrogen for one to five years resulted in a threefold increase in uterine cancer.

- Use of unopposed estrogen for ten years resulted in about a tenfold increase in uterine cancer.
- Lifetime use of unopposed estrogen could increase the risk even higher—to about one in ten users.
- The increased risk lingered after stopping estrogen, with about a twofold increase persisting for about five years.
- Deaths from uterine cancer were increased two- to threefold.

Before any more fear sets in, permit me to place things in perspective.

- Uterine cancer is not particularly common, occurring in about 1 in 1,000 women each year.
- Uterine cancer caused by unopposed estrogen was less invasive and had a much higher overall cure rate (more than 90 percent) than uterine cancer in general (about 70 to 75 percent).
- Doctors don't use unopposed estrogen any longer—unless a woman has had a hysterectomy.
- Adding progesterone to estrogen *erases* any increased risk.

Lessons from Biology I: The Importance of Progesterone

In the first half of the menstrual cycle, while the egg is being developed, estrogen is being manufactured by the ovary. In the last half of the cycle—just after the egg has been released—the ovary also secretes progesterone (pro = in favor of, gest = gestation = pregnancy). Progesterone changes the uterine lining to make it ready for pregnancy. If no pregnancy occurs, progesterone production stops after about two weeks, the uterine lining sheds, and the cycle begins again.

Even in nature, progesterone is added to estrogen. As always, it's best to stand in awe of nature's genius and do your best to mimic it. What we have learned, painfully, is that progesterone is necessary to keep the growth-promoting effects of estrogen in check. We need to replace *both* hormones.

Estrogen causes uterine cells to divide. Progesterone inhibits this growth. Progesterone does this in several ways:

- Progesterone reduces estrogen receptors in the cell—making the cell less responsive to estrogen.
- Progesterone encourages the cell to convert the *type* of estrogen from the stronger estradiol to the weaker estrone.
- Progesterone helps prevent the estrogen receptor from stimulating cancer-promoting genes.

When women don't ovulate, they don't produce progesterone. Some women don't ovulate for many years, and unfortunately these women *do* suffer from an increased risk of uterine cancer. More commonly, however, these women develop a less serious overgrowth of the uterine lining called *hyperplasia* (hyper = over, plasia = growth). However, this lesion can become more significantly precancerous when the nuclei of the cells become abnormal and atypical. In this case, the lesion is called *atypical hyperplasia*. Perhaps 15 to 25 percent of women with atypical hyperplasia will progress to uterine cancer if left untreated.

Lessons from Biology II: Progesterone Prevents Pre-Malignant Changes

In a landmark study, Dr. J. Donald Woodruff and The Menopause Study Group carefully and extensively studied the effects of four different estrogen-progesterone regimens compared to a fifth regimen consisting of estrogen alone. Each group consisted of about 275 women. All women in every group received 0.625 mg of conjugated estrogens every day. The groups were divided as follows:

Two groups received progesterone for fourteen days a month (at 5 mg and 10 mg doses).

Two groups received progesterone daily (at 2.5 mg and 5 mg doses).

One group received *only* Premarin, 0.625 mg daily (*no* progesterone added).

The study continued for one year with striking and informative results:

- 20 percent of women on estrogen alone developed a weakly premalignant form of hyperplasia after one year.
- None of the regimens containing progesterone caused more than a 1 percent incidence of hyperplasia (which is considered normal).
- The two regimens with higher-dose progesterone (10 mg daily for fourteen days of each month, or 5 mg every day) had *zero* incidence of hyperplasia.

This study confirms two fundamental facts. First, unopposed estrogen leads to an abnormal uterine lining in a significant percentage of women. Second, the addition of progesterone reduces the risk to at least normal baseline levels, or perhaps to a level *below* baseline risk (a *protective* effect). This zero incidence of hyperplasia at the higher progesterone doses confirms earlier studies (albeit much smaller) by Nachtigall and Hammond that also reported a zero incidence of uterine cancer, and corresponds with the 80 percent reduction in uterine cancer reported by Gambrell (also a much smaller study).

In essence, the ability of progesterone to reduce the occurrence of abnormal uterine changes to normal or below-normal levels is certainly in line with the notion that *estrogen with progesterone added causes no increase in uterine cancer and may actually be protective*. However, a few cautionary notes:

- The incidence of uterine cancer while taking estrogen-progesterone will *not* be zero. For example, though *rare*, there have been reports of uterine cancer occurring in women who were taking daily estrogen-progesterone (as reported by Comerci and colleagues).
- Simply lowering the dose of unopposed estrogen to 0.3 mg per day will *not* work. A fivefold increased rate of cancer was reported by Cushing and colleagues at this dose.
- Progesterone must be taken for at least *ten* days a month. There is still some debate about whether it should be ten, twelve, or fourteen days, but most clinicians are happy with ten days. Some early reports regarding the use of progesterone fourteen days every two months or even three months so far reveal a good safety profile (about a 1 percent annual incidence of hyperplasia).

Estrogen Use in Uterine Cancer Survivors

Clinicians are far more comfortable with estrogen-replacement therapy in women following the treatment of uterine cancer as opposed to breast cancer. Following several reports suggesting that estrogen-replacement therapy could be used safely following treatment for uterine cancer, the 1990 committee opinion of the American College of Obstetricians and Gynecologists stated that, "For women with a history of (uterine) cancer, *estrogen could be used for the same indications as for any other woman,* except that the selection of appropriate candidates should be based upon prognostic indicators and the risk the patient is willing to assume. The need to treat . . . may outweigh the risk of stimulating tumor growth."

Given the fact that there are 36,000 new uterine cancers diagnosed annually in the United States, with the largest number of patients between the ages of fifty and fifty-nine, this issue is especially important. About 75 percent of patients present as Stage I disease with an excellent cure rate. In fact, the risk of recurrence for early-stage disease may be as low as 0 to 3 percent. As stated by Dr. Julia Chapman,

> Many survivors of uterine cancer have significant menopausal symptoms and other illnesses directly related to estrogen deprivation after therapy for the cancer. The literature supports the use of menopausal estrogens for the relief of the menopausal syndrome and for the prevention of postmenopausal osteoporosis and cardiovascular disease, both of which result in a mortality rate that exceeds that of uterine cancer.

Concluding Thoughts

There is no question that the increased incidence of uterine cancer resulting from the use of unopposed estrogen in the 1960s, and publicized in the 1970s, released a shock wave from which both doctors and patients have been slow to recover.

On this point, however, the data are abundantly clear. The addition of growth-inhibiting progesterone does indeed provide protection against any increased risk of uterine cancer. It is also highly likely that, if any abnormality begins to develop, modern diagnostic technology, such as ultrasound and (a now more gentle) uterine biopsy, would likely provide early diagnosis leading to early intervention and cure.

In my judgment, the relationship between uterine cancer and hormone-replacement therapy is now one *less* barrier that should stand between women and the benefits of estrogen.

Key Points to Consider

- Estrogen use *with* progesterone added almost certainly does not increase the incidence of uterine cancer. In fact, there is strong scientific data to support the notion that women on estrogen and progesterone will actually develop fewer cases of uterine cancer than woman who don't take hormones at all.

- Estrogen alone (without progesterone) can lead to an abnormal uterine lining in a significant percentage of women.

6

THE PERKS:
How Estrogen Improves the Quality of Life

Unlike the highly charged debate about estrogen and breast cancer, the ability of hormone-replacement therapy to relieve bothersome symptoms of menopause and maintain youthfulness is widely acknowledged. In fact, the prevention and relief of menopausal symptoms such as hot flashes is the main reason why many women *start* taking estrogen—and then *stop* taking it a few years later when they perceive it's no longer needed.

In this book, I have sought to reverse this perception. Estrogen is actually needed lifelong for the prevention of heart disease, osteoporosis, and Alzheimer's disease. That estrogen also provides for better *quality* of life and better sex should really be considered "the perks" of using hormone replacement.

Many of these benefits have already been touched upon. Improvements of mood and memory, and indeed a global sense of well-being were reviewed in the chapter on the brain. Beneficial effects on glucose metabolism and diabetes were discussed in the heart chapter, as was the prevention of strokes. Better balance demonstrated by estrogen users was discussed in the bones chapter as an additional mechanism of fracture prevention.

Issues which directly impact upon the quality of life, such as hot flashes, sleep disturbance, and sexual difficulties, will be discussed here. We will also explore estrogen's effects upon the urinary tract, skin, and fat distribution, as well as its possible effects on colon cancer and rheumatoid arthritis.

The Classic Hot Flash

It's a well-known fact that estrogen relieves hot flashes. Hot flashes affect the large majority of menopausal women. Estimates vary: anywhere from 75 percent to more than 90 percent are affected, with at least 10 to 15 percent of women considering the problem to be severe. Studies calculate that about four million women in the United States are currently severely affected, such that their daily living is disrupted. Though dosage adjustments may be necessary, hormone-replacement therapy cures at least 80 percent (a bit conservative) to nearly 100 percent (more likely) of patients.

In general, hot flashes continue for six months to two years. However, in as many as 25 percent of women, they persist for longer than five years. In some patients, they can continue for ten or twenty years or longer. Obese women tend to have milder symptoms, no doubt due to the ability of fat cells to convert various hormones to estrogen. Conversely, smokers tend to have somewhat more severe symptoms due to the anti-estrogen effects of cigarette smoke.

Variability of symptoms is striking. The onset of hot flashes varies from the premenopausal years to several years after menopause, though the latter is uncommon. The frequency of hot flashes also varies widely and for no observable reason. Hot flashes can occur many times daily or only once in a while and even this pattern often changes. A hot flash itself typically lasts from three to six minutes, with both shorter and longer durations reported.

It is the *decline* of estrogen from previously normal levels, rather than the low level itself, that causes hot flashes. Abrupt changes in estrogen levels, such as occurs when the ovaries are surgically removed from premenopausal women, generally cause more severe symptoms. In fact, hot flashes have occurred in *men* when their testicles have been removed surgically, generating an abrupt drop in testosterone—and estrogen—levels.

The Mechanism of a Hot Flash

In an area of the brain called the *hypothalamus* are nerve cells that regulate the body's temperature. These nerve cells have estrogen receptors and are directly influenced by estrogen. When estrogen levels decline, the temperature regulatory centers of the hypothalamus are disturbed and cease to function normally. Think of this as a thermostat at home with which people tamper. In the typical American family, one member lowers the thermostat and some time later someone else grouchily puts it back in its original place.

In a woman's body, a hot flash is set in motion when the "thermostat" is placed at a lower setting. The body then tries to cool down to this lower temperature setting by *releasing heat*. In this attempt, the body sends blood from the inner core to the outer surface (the skin) to cool down. To facilitate the cool-down, blood vessels near the surface of the body widen (causing the flush), the heart rate quickens (palpitations), and skin temperature rises by 10 to 15 degrees (causing the feeling of intense heat). Ultimately the body perspires. At this point the thermostat is raised back to its original setting. The body must now seek to raise its temperature by *conserving* heat. Often the body shivers in an attempt to create heat and this can be accompanied by a sensation of a chill. At the same time, the peripheral blood vessels constrict in order to return blood to the inner core of the body, diminishing the flush and returning the skin to its normal color.

The opening and closing of the blood vessels, transferring blood from the inner core of the body to the skin and back, gives the hot flash its medical term: "vasomotor instability" (vaso = blood vessel, motor = contracting and dilating).

Many women have a premonition of an impending hot flash—an *aura*—often described as a tingling sensation in the hands and scalp, pressure in the head, along with a sense of anxiety. Though the level of severity is often described as mild, nobody seems to have anything good to say about hot flashes. Consequently, I would simply suggest that you take estrogen in a timely manner, leave the thermostat where it is, and happily avoid the whole problem.

Sleep Disturbance

Estrogen receptors have been found in regions of the brain responsible for sleep regulation, such as the hypothalamus, the preoptic area, and the hippocampus. Estrogen may also affect sleep by altering the levels of neurotransmitters—including acetylcholine and dopamine, as well as serotonin—which play a role in regulating sleep patterns.

Erlik and others used EEG (electro-encephalogram, for brain-wave analysis) and skin-temperature measurements to show that postmenopausal women who awoke suddenly during the night did so as a result of hot flashes that occurred during sleep. Shaver and colleagues showed that the quality of sleep is poorer, as measured by the amount of REM (rapid eye movement) sleep in women with hot flashes compared to those who have no hot flashes.

"Night sweats" are hot flashes that occur during sleep, but in fact, falling estrogen levels can cause sleep disruption even if night sweats are not present. Sleep deprivation as a result of nighttime hot flashes can contribute to the daytime fatigue, mood swings, and irritability that have been so closely linked with menopause.

Studies show that women who take estrogen fall asleep more easily and stay asleep longer with fewer periods of wakefulness. Estrogen improves sleep patterns *directly* by its effect on brain function, and *indirectly* by relieving debilitating physical symptoms and mood disturbance, which can themselves lead to sleep disturbance. Estrogen's direct effect on the brain is strongly supported by the fact that even women who don't suffer any other menopausal symptoms sleep better if they're taking estrogen.

Vaginal Changes

The tissues that line the entire genitourinary tract are richly endowed with estrogen receptors and are greatly affected by declining estrogen levels. With the loss of estrogen, the vaginal walls get progressively thinner. They lose the elasticity and resilience they had when estrogen was prominent and the vagina itself becomes shorter and narrower. The medical term for this process is, unfortunately, "vaginal atrophy"—and the fact is, eventually it happens to most women.

As they thin out, the vaginal walls can sometimes diminish to only a few cells thick, from their normal thickness of about fifty cells. Not only are the numbers of cells reduced, but a certain *type* of cells—namely the "superficial cells," which are rich in glycogen (a natural sugar)—becomes nearly absent altogether. These superficial cells, especially when supported by good blood flow, secrete glycogen, which becomes food for healthy vaginal bacteria—the lactobacilli.

The growth of these helpful bacteria, supported by vaginal glycogen, releases lactic acid, which creates an acidic environment hostile to any invading, opportunistic, or harmful organisms. When estrogen production stops, the acid balance of the vagina slowly shifts away from acidic and toward a more alkaline environment. This makes the vagina more hospitable to hostile bacteria. Dryness and subsequent irritation make vaginal tissues vulnerable to infection as well. Some reports state that the prevalence of this "atrophic vaginitis" affects up to 38 percent of postmenopausal women.

In the absence of estrogen, blood flow to the genitals decreases. So it takes longer to produce lubrication in preparation for intercourse. Vaginal lubrication diminishes as well because low levels of circulating estrogen no longer stimulate the production of cervical and vaginal mucus. Some lubrication may still be derived from small amounts of estrogen still remaining in the body and from the Bartholin's glands, small glands located at the entrance of the vagina.

These physical changes can make sex uncomfortable, painful, or even impossible. As many as 30 percent of postmenopausal women complain of painful intercourse and consequently have sex less often. This is unfortunate, because having sex *increases* the blood flow to tissues, encourages the production of mucous secretions, helps to maintain muscle tone, and preserves the shape and size of the vagina. Still, even sexually active women may eventually have the same problem other women have unless they use estrogen.

All in all, by several mechanisms, estrogen therapy promotes and maintains the physical and sexual functioning of the vagina. Estrogen increases blood flow to the vagina, builds up vaginal lining to a healthy state, and increases vaginal lubrication for women with a particularly thin and fragile vaginal lining. In the presence of estrogen, the normal acidic environment will return, as will a more normal resistance to infection. Though it may take several months, and even up to a year, for complete restoration of normal anatomy and function, a more pleasurable sex life is often enjoyed in a matter of a few weeks.

However, the problem can be avoided entirely by the timely use of estrogen.

Sexuality

In a study of women aged fifty to eighty-two in Madison, Wisconsin, nearly one-half reported an ongoing sexual relationship. Likewise, in the Duke Longitudinal Study on Aging, 50 percent of all older women were still interested in sex. In the same study, however, 70 percent of men were sexually active and 80 percent reported interest in sexual activity. Though these contrasting figures may represent cultural factors, the relative stability of hormone levels in aging men compared to the decreasing levels in menopausal women may also be relevant.

As stated by Dr. Barbara Sherwin,* human sexual behavior comprises two distinct but interrelated processes, *libido* and *potency*. Libido refers to sexual desire, sexual fantasies, and satisfaction or pleasure. Potency refers to increased blood flow and resultant swelling of tissues, (pelvic vasocongestion), orgasmic contractions, and other bodily aspects of sexual response.

It is clear that estrogen deprivation affects the physical aspects of a woman's sexual functioning, or potency. As was previously discussed, vaginal changes such as decreased lubrication, increased infection, and anatomic changes including the shortening and narrowing of the vagina can lead to painful intercourse. In addition, the reduced blood flow to the reproductive tissues leads to decreased vasocongestion, which can also lead to de-

*Dr. Sherwin cites the work of J. M. Davidson.

creased lubrication as well as decreased sensation. Fortunately, these physical changes that impact negatively on a woman's sexuality are *quite reliably* prevented and reversed by estrogen administration.

When physical difficulties impair sexual functioning, concern, anxiety, and diminished pleasure can affect both partners—leading not only to diminished sexual activity (which, unfortunately, only makes matters worse for vaginal tissues), but also to decreased interest in sex. By ameliorating the physical difficulties and preventing this downward spiral, estrogen *indirectly* improves libido, no doubt aided by estrogen's additional beneficial effects on mood and psychological well-being.

A *direct* effect on libido—the motivational aspects of sexual behavior, including desire and fantasies—clearly appears to be the province of *testosterone.* Fortunately, the decrease in testosterone at menopause is not nearly as profound as the decrease in estrogen. In fact, in natural menopause the decrease in circulating testosterone is only about 15 to 25 percent. (After surgical removal of the ovaries, the decrease in testosterone is significantly more pronounced.)

Luckily, the ovary is not a woman's only source of testosterone. In fact, the ovary produces only 25 percent of circulating testosterone. Other sources of testosterone are the adrenal glands and the conversion by the body of other androgenic hormones (andro = male, genic = to generate) into testosterone. In addition, the postmenopausal ovary continues to secrete significant, if not increased, amounts of testosterone. Thus, even though circulating testosterone levels are lower at menopause, this reduction is not necessarily associated with decreased libido in menopausal women.

There is absolutely no question that testosterone supplementation enhances libido. Many studies of postmenopausal women complaining of decreased libido reported a superior response to testosterone-containing regimens when compared to regimens of estrogen alone. The immediate cautionary note to be sounded, however, is that testosterone use may carry a price tag. Namely, it might impair some of estrogen's beneficial, life-saving effects on cholesterol levels and heart disease. (I will go into this in greater detail in Chapter 7.)

Urinary Problems

Studies indicate that up to 40 percent of menopausal women have some form of urinary leakage, which is called urinary incontinence. Similar numbers of women complain of frequent urination, a sudden urge to urinate (even though the bladder is not full), and occasional painful urination. Making matters worse, fewer than half of incontinent women seek help—often because of embarrassment or the misconception that the condition is an inevitable consequence of aging.

Urinary tract tissues in women are embryologically related to the genital tract. Estrogen receptors have been identified in the urethra and bladder, as well as in the muscles of the pelvis. Just as with the lining of the vagina, with menopause, the lining of the urethra may become thin, and the surrounding muscles and elastic tissues may weaken. Estrogen has been shown to enhance the tone of the urethra, allowing it to increase its pressure (think of the urethra as a straw squeezing itself shut) and hold back any undesired flow of urine from the bladder. Estrogen also allows the blood vessels in the urethra to become more swollen (from improved blood flow), which somewhat helps compress the urethra to keep it closed. Given these findings and the known association of the postmenopausal years with increased urinary tract problems, it has been widely assumed that estrogen loss plays a major role in the development of these problems—and that its replacement will cure them.

Estrogen-replacement therapy does ease some urinary symptoms, but it stops well short of a cure. Though a substantial proportion of patients with urinary problems who take estrogen feel better when you measure their bladder function in a laboratory, estrogen users are *not* significantly different from nonusers. Why, then, are *symptoms* relieved by estrogen?

One idea is that estrogen makes the bladder less sensitive to stimuli. Without estrogen, the bladder may overreact with increased contractions—creating an urge to urinate, or leading to an increased frequency of urination, especially at night. "Nocturia" (noct = nocturnal), can be particularly bothersome. By decreasing the sensitivity and "hyper" functioning of the bladder, there is less disruption of daily living.

Another mechanism by which estrogen provides improvement is the prevention of urinary tract infections (which also cause a frequent urge to urinate). Unlike other urinary problems, the ability of estrogen to prevent these infections in menopausal women has unequivocal scientific support. Estrogen users have significantly fewer urinary tract infections, presumably because estrogen returns the vaginal environment to its original state, encouraging the return of lactobacilli, and removing the offending bacteria. Indeed, compared to nonusers, many estrogen users remain free of urinary tract infection.

In sum, regarding the urinary tract, estrogen may best be considered a role player, providing supportive therapy and improving comfort level. Still, all urinary complaints should receive prompt and expert attention. Proper diagnosis and individualized treatment—which may be a combination of medical, surgical, and behavioral therapy—is essential.

Skin

In general, as people age, their skin-cell replacement slows down, as does the elastic fiber content. As a result, the skin becomes drier, thinner, less elastic, and more inclined to wrinkle. In women, it has been shown that skin collagen and skin thickness steadily decrease with time after menopause. Women can lose up to 30 percent of skin collagen in the first five years following menopause. Happily, this decrease is *prevented* by hormone-replacement therapy. The fact that collagen loss accelerates during the first several years after menopause suggests that if supplemental estrogens do indeed benefit skin, it might be best to begin therapy early.

Also of considerable importance is the natural diminishing of the layer of fat cells of the skin. This subcutaneous fat provides inner support, firmness, and resilience to the skin. Estrogen helps maintain this layer by stimulating the production of hyaluronic acid, which holds water and maintains the moisture of the tissues.

In the first randomized, double-blind, placebo-controlled study addressing the effects of estrogen-replacement therapy on skin thickness, a 1994 Canadian study evaluated sixty postmenopausal nuns (aged fifty-one to seventy-one) whose limited exposure to sun and smoking provided a clearer reading of what changing hormone levels themselves could do to skin. After twelve months of taking estrogen, those in the treated group showed a 30 percent *increase* in the thickness of the dermis (the inner layer of the skin), and an 11.5 percent *increase* in overall skin thickness. No significant skin changes were observed in the placebo group.

Similar studies found that estrogen can inhibit the loss of skin collagen and thickness within six months, and can even restore a substantial amount of what was lost. *There is also some indication that as skin thickness increases, wrinkling might be reduced.* However, once a certain threshold is reached, long-term hormone use does not appear to have any further effect on skin.

Weight Gain

Since everybody *thinks* that estrogen causes weight gain, let me state an accepted fact: *Estrogen therapy doesn't cause an ounce of weight gain.*

A study of five hundred postmenopausal women by Judith Wurtman at the Massachusetts Institute of Technology revealed that 64 percent of nonobese women gained an average of ten to fifteen pounds after menopause. Obese menopausal women fared even more poorly—94 percent gained an average of twenty-one to twenty-three pounds after menopause. When estrogen replacement was factored into the equation—that is, when women taking estrogen were measured against women *not* taking estrogen, there was *no* difference in weight gain. In fact, in most studies (seven of eleven by one count) the hormone users actually weighed slightly *less*.

Still another "perk" estrogen users enjoy involves fat distribution. It appears estrogen is responsible for keeping a woman's fat in the right places. Scientists call this "gynecoid fat distribution," measured by the waist-to-hip ratio. Estrogen users maintain a more favorable waist-to-hip ratio (less waist, more hip), whereas nonusers begin after menopause to redistribute their fat to the waist and abdomen, attaining a more "android" fat distribution somewhat reminiscent of their spouses, or yours truly.

Tooth Loss

Tooth loss, like osteoporosis, accelerates in women (but not in men) after age fifty. Women who have osteoporosis need dentures far more frequently than women who do not have osteoporosis. In one study, Dr. H. W. Daniell showed that among women with osteoporosis who still had their natural teeth at age fifty, 44 percent required a full denture by age sixty, compared to only 15 percent of women who did not have osteoporosis. Dr. Daniell went on to theorize that bone loss can occur *before* gum disease and cause the loss of teeth. He also showed that black women, who are less prone to develop osteoporosis, had much less loss of oral bone, and much less gum disease as a result. It stands to reason, then, that estrogen use, by preventing osteoporosis, will also prevent bone loss in the oral cavity and the resultant periodontal disease and loss of teeth.

Rheumatoid Arthritis

There is a scientific argument going on as to whether estrogen use, or even oral contraceptive use in younger women, affects the development or clinical severity of rheumatoid arthritis. Studies from the Netherlands, which have concentrated on patients with severe forms of the disease, showed that oral contraceptive use in premenopausal women and estrogen-replacement therapy in postmenopausal women decreased the incidence and severity of rheumatoid arthritis. But two other studies, one of which was done at the Mayo Clinic, found *no* underlying effect. The rebuttal from the Netherlands was that the patients they studied had more severe symptoms, which made it easier to tell when these symptoms were decreased.

It would certainly be nice to think that estrogen's known ability to help regulate the immune system and keep inflammatory chemicals in check—mechanisms by which estrogen may prevent Alzheimer's disease—could lead to significant improvement of rheumatoid arthritis, but this may not be the case. However, there may still be some patients for whom estrogen use provides some degree of improvement.

Colon Cancer

There is new and accumulating evidence that current users and, to a lesser extent, past users of estrogen have about a 35 percent decrease in the risk of developing colon cancer. Three large studies used a prospective approach, following a large group of women—estrogen users and nonusers—for several years. Results of all three studies showed that estrogen use afforded a 22 to 45 percent decrease in onset of the disease. In addition, most studies showed a decrease in adenomatous polyps, which arise in the colon and are thought to be precancerous. However, the studies show a significant benefit only while women are taking estrogen.

As regards colon cancer, estrogen's protective effects work in the following ways:

- Bile acids can cause the lining cells of the colon to grow and possibly initiate malignant change. Estrogen decreases bile acids.
- Certain bacteria digest the bile acids and then excrete a chemical (diacylglycerol) which can initiate malignant change. Estrogen may directly decrease the population of these bacteria by decreasing the bacteria's bile-acid food supply, resulting in a greatly reduced production of the harmful cancer-producing chemical.
- Colon-lining cells with a full complement of estrogen receptors seem less prone to malignant change. Estrogen receptors may bind to harmful chemicals before these chemicals have a chance to bind to more dangerous parts of the cell's DNA.

It is estimated by the authors of the Nurses Health Study that estrogen use may decrease the yearly rate of colon cancer development from 8 cases to 5 per 10,000 in women aged fifty-five to fifty-nine, and from 12 cases to 6 per 10,000 women aged sixty to sixty-four. Given the quality of the research and its theoretical underpinnings, these calculations are most encouraging.

Key Points to Consider

► It's a well-known fact that estrogen relieves hot flashes. Hot flashes affect a large majority of menopausal women. It is estimated that from 75 percent to more than 90 percent are affected, with at least 10 to 15 percent of women considering the problem to be severe.

► Regarding sleep disturbance: Studies show that women who take estrogen fall asleep more easily and stay asleep longer with fewer periods of wakefulness.

► As many as 30 percent of postmenopausal women complain of painful intercourse and consequently have sex less often. The timely use of estrogen can prevent the vaginal changes that cause these problems. Irritating symptoms can be alleviated by estrogen use within a matter of weeks, but may take up to a year to disappear entirely depending on the situation.

► By ameliorating physical sexual difficulties, estrogen *indirectly* improves libido, no doubt aided by estrogen's additional beneficial effects on mood and psychological well-being.

► There is no question that testosterone supplementation enhances libido in many patients.

► Studies indicate that up to 40 percent of menopausal women have urinary incontinence. Similar numbers of women complain of frequent and/or painful urination. Estrogen-replacement therapy does ease some urinary symptoms—

including preventing urinary tract infections and making the bladder less sensitive to stimuli—but it stops well short of a cure.

- ▶ Estrogen can inhibit the loss of skin collagen and thickness within six months, and can even restore a substantial amount of what was lost. There is also some indication that as skin thickness increases, wrinkling might be reduced.

- ▶ Estrogen therapy does not cause an ounce of weight gain.

- ▶ Tooth loss, like osteoporosis, accelerates in women (but not in men) after age fifty. Estrogen use, by preventing osteoporosis, will also prevent bone loss in the oral cavity and the resultant periodontal disease and loss of teeth.

- ▶ There is new and accumulating evidence that current users and, to a lesser extent, past users of estrogen have about a 35 percent decrease in the risk of developing colon cancer.

7

HORMONE REGIMENS AND SIDE EFFECTS:

An Overview

Only about 20 percent of women take hormone replacement long-term. If even a small portion of the other 80 percent were on any reasonable hormone regime, countless lives could be saved. When doctors prescribe other medications, generally 50 to 90 percent of patients comply and continue treatment. Such is not the case with hormones, however. In the first place, 50 percent of women don't even fill their prescriptions. And of those who do, no more than 25 percent continue hormone replacement long-term.

Among the reasons cited by women for dismissing hormones are fear of cancer, concern about side effects, and the fact that they don't believe they need them.

Women's noncompliance with hormone-replacement therapy can't be about side effects, though. Other drugs have side effects, and both men and women continue taking them. Rather, it seems women don't take estrogen because they don't think estrogen is *good* for them. I believe if women become convinced of the profound overall benefits of estrogen replacement—and perceive a need to take it—tolerance and acceptance of any side effects will not be a problem. In fact, studies show that, overall, menopausal women *feel better* on estrogen.

Nonetheless, hormones are *not* all equal in terms of how they work or the side effects they produce. Because each woman responds to medication in her own way, it is important to understand the various options available before decisions are made. There is no question that therapy should be individualized. Therefore, an ongoing dialogue between patient and physician is essential.

Today, hormone-replacement regimens can be tailored to your personal needs—you and your physician can select the regimen that offers the most benefit while minimizing side effects. Doses may need to be adjusted over time, however, because often the first choice of medication is not as successful as we'd like.

What matters most is that you take it.

Replacement of Hormones versus Relief of Symptoms

Oral and transdermal (the patch) estrogens are used for hormone-replacement therapy, and are the only routes of administration that provide access to estrogen's life-saving benefits. Estrogen in other forms, such as vaginal cream and the new estrogen "ring," is useful only at combating local symptoms such as vaginal dryness, some urinary complaints, and painful intercourse. To further complicate matters, a new "low dose" patch provides slightly more estrogen to reduce hot flashes, but is not adequate to provide the full benefits of hormone replacement.

Estrogen-Replacement Regimens: Issues and Options

Oral is better. The story dates back to the late 1970s, when estrogen was still trying to escape out from under the two dark clouds with which it had been associated—uterine cancer and blood clots. As we have previously discussed, the risk of uterine cancer was largely eliminated when it was learned that giving progesterone would counter estrogen's effects on the uterus. But at that time there had not yet been an answer to the problem of blood clots. (This was also before we knew that blood clots resulted from too strong a dose of birth-control pills.) Ciba-Geigy designed an estrogen patch that could be placed directly on the skin. As such, the estrogen did not travel first to the liver ("first pass") because it was not being swallowed and placed into the digestive tract.

It was felt that by *avoiding* the liver (which manufactures clotting factors), there would be no increase in these factors and, therefore, the patch would cause fewer problems with blood clots. In essence, it was felt the patch would be safer and ultimately preferable. Alas, such is not the case at all.

It turns out we *want* estrogen to go to the liver. It is in the liver where estrogen exerts its effects, such as increasing the level of the "good" HDL cholesterol, and decreasing the "bad" LDL cholesterol. Transdermal estrogen does *not* increase the level of the important HDL-2 cholesterol to anywhere near the 30 to 40 percent increase that oral estrogen accomplishes. Transdermal estrogen increases total HDL cholesterol by only 1 or 2 percent—perhaps up to 5 percent—compared to the 13 to 17 percent increase found with oral estrogen. Given the fact that these changes in cholesterol levels account for one-quarter to one-half of estrogen's protective effect against heart disease, I'd stay with oral estrogen and avoid the patch.

Even the idea that the patch is better for avoiding blood clots doesn't hold up entirely. First of all, no one has ever proven that the patch causes less clotting (which, I remind you, is *not* an overwhelming threat in the first place—with an incidence of about 1 in 10,000). Second, oral estrogen causes a 50 percent *reduction* of a circulating chemical (PAI-1) that can cause blood clots. Transdermal estrogen has no such effect.

It should be noted, however, that the patch does *not* increase triglyceride levels to the same extent as oral estrogen. Consequently, the use of the patch is recommended by many experts for patients who have elevated triglyceride levels. Unless there is a digestive problem, or some other special reason, the rest of the world should use oral estrogen.

*Types of Oral Estrogen**

What type of oral estrogen should you use? Once again, given the current state of affairs, where most women worldwide are not taking estrogen, the simple answer is, *it doesn't make any difference.* What *is* true is that some

*"Designer" estrogens (SERMS) are discussed in the next chapter.

women feel better taking one type of estrogen as opposed to another—so physician and patient should be open-minded and willing to adjust as necessary.

That said, what follows is a brief listing and accompanying commentary regarding the available estrogen formulations.

CONJUGATED ESTROGENS (PREMARIN)

Conjugated estrogens are the most widely studied of all estrogen formulations, even though the relative importance of all their ingredients is still not fully understood. Premarin has been available since 1941 and is a compilation of seventeen to twenty estrogen-like substances extracted from the urine of pregnant mares. Historically, before scientists had the ability to synthesize hormones precisely, they were able to extract hormones from animal tissues. Premarin has undergone years of rigorous scientific evaluation—and has quite successfully withstood the test of time.

ESTRADIOL (ESTRACE)

Estradiol is different from conjugated estrogen because it is fully synthesized in a laboratory. Some consider it to be closer to "natural" because it is identical to a woman's estradiol. But "natural" is a term that is deceiving. Most women don't realize estradiol is only *one* form of estrogen. In a woman's body, there are actually *three* different estrogens: estradiol, estrone, and estriol. Estradiol is the most powerful. Over the course of a woman's lifetime, and indeed during the course of a menstrual cycle, the relative amounts of these estrogens change.

ESTRONE (OGEN, ORTHO-EST)

Estrone is the dominant circulating estrogen in menopausal women. Therefore, a notion arose that its use was metabolically more appropriate than using estradiol or other formulations. However, *no* apparent clinical difference has been found when estrone is used in equivalent doses.

ESTERIFIED ESTROGENS (ESTRATAB)

These are derived from plant sources (hopefully from a plant with a favorable waist-to-hip ratio). The drug company's advertisement shows a picture of various plants, complete with text referring to "a natural decision . . . rooted in nature." This is what the world is coming to. If every postmenopausal woman mysteriously piled yams high on her plate, or wandered off into the fields to chew on soy leaves, I'd say the company was on to something. Failing that, this more distinctly resembles an idea born "naturally" in a Madison Avenue hatchery. Regardless, esterified estrogens have not been as extensively studied and they do not seem to have any clinically distinguishing features.

Choice of Progesterone or Progestin

When discussing estrogen and the prevention of heart disease, I mentioned that there were essentially three groups of hormones colloquially known as "progesterone," some form of which a woman must take along with estrogen.*

*For a detailed discussion of progesterone please see pages 49–51.

Of these, "natural" progesterone and Provera (a "weak" progestin) should be considered. The group of "strong" progestins, such as Norethindrone—which are also used in birth control pills—is more widely used in Europe for hormone replacement. I personally do *not* recommend their use because of metabolic side effects, such as a particularly unfavorable impact on HDL and LDL cholesterol levels. Clinical practice has shifted toward the use of the following two formulations:

PROVERA

I use this particular brand name first because few people recognize its chemical name, medroxyprogesterone acetate. The use of this form of progesterone has successfully withstood extensive testing over time. There has been some concern regarding the slight diminution of estrogen's positive effects on cholesterol levels with the use of Provera. However, *no* reduction of estrogen's beneficial effects on heart disease has been found.

MICRONIZED PROGESTERONE

This is the same progesterone that is manufactured by the ovary. As such, it is indeed natural. Hormones in their "natural" form have only recently been able to be given orally. Unless broken down into small particles (micronized), natural hormones will be digested and rendered ineffective. Since the successful use of this micronizing process is relatively recent, we still have much to learn about this form of progesterone. Some recent studies have implied that micronized progesterone may be preferable to Provera because of a more favorable effect on cholesterol levels, but other studies have shown *no* difference. In addition, micronized progesterone does not cause vasospasm of arteries, which has occurred with Provera. Whether there is any chemical difference between these two formulations remains to be seen.

Cyclic versus Daily Regimens

Cyclic versus daily treatment is entirely a matter of personal preference. However, it does seem to be increasingly apparent that, by the time they become menopausal, most women do not feel the need to continue to menstruate. A daily dose of estrogen combined with progesterone can accomplish this. The problem is that clinical reality comes up far short of early expectations. Especially in the first two years after menopause, far fewer (only 50 to 80 percent) than the hoped-for 90 percent of women stop bleeding after six to twelve months of daily therapy. Therefore, some degree of trial and error is necessary. Daily therapy is most successful after the first or second year of menopause. (Prior to that, cyclic therapy may be necessary to avoid breakthrough bleeding in some women.)

Cyclic regimens mimic a menstrual cycle and consist of daily estrogen to which is added ten to fourteen days a month of progesterone. After progesterone is stopped, "progesterone withdrawal bleeding" (similar to a period) occurs. In some women, this bleeding diminishes over time and completely ceases. In others it persists for years. It often turns out that, after one or two years of cyclic therapy, women can successfully switch to daily therapy.

One newer alternative technique combines aspects of both regimens. Namely, daily estrogen and progesterone are continued from days 1 to 25. Predictable bleeding occurs on days 26 to 27 and may well be preferred by some patients.

I am not aware of *any* data revealing a remarkable difference between regimens or choice of hormones. Rather, it is far more important for women to partake of any one of the accepted regimens. While there is no question that the various tissues of a woman's body have different reactions to estrogen, the accepted dose range of conjugated estrogens (and estrone) is 0.625 mg to 1.25 mg daily. This is equivalent to 1 mg to 2 mg of estradiol daily, or 0.05 mg to 0.1 mg of daily estradiol via transdermal patches replaced once or twice weekly. Many of estrogen's protective effects (particularly on bone) are lost when the dose falls below these minimal levels. For some intolerant patients, however, suboptimal doses probably provide some beneficial effect.

I have no qualms with the prudent recommendation that the "minimum effective dose" of estrogen be used. However, I do not think a woman should needlessly suffer hot flashes when an increased dose would provide relief. In addition, there is now early data suggesting that higher doses of estrogen provide greater degrees of protection against Alzheimer's disease. These benefits might ultimately outweigh suggestions from breast cancer studies that we should minimize estrogen doses. Once again, doctor and patient will have to sort this out together.

Less-than-Monthly Use of Progesterone

This regimen may well represent a viable alternative for those women intolerant of progestins or those who prefer less than monthly bleeding. Two studies using Provera at a dose of 10 mg for fourteen days every three months ("quarterly progesterone") were performed by Ettinger and Williams. Both studies revealed an acceptable safety profile. The Ettinger study reported that, even though the bleeding was somewhat heavier (seven versus five days) compared to that with monthly progesterone, the women preferred the quarterly regimen by a ratio of 4 to 1. There was some concern that less-than-monthly progesterone might not provide an adequate degree of protection against the development of abnormal uterine cells. Fortunately, the 1.5 percent incidence of uterine hyperplasia was not much different from the expected 1 percent incidence.

On Giving Estrogen After Hysterectomy and Surgical Removal of the Ovaries

Young women who have surgical menopause have hot flashes that are more severe and last far longer—an average of 8.5 years—than women undergoing natural menopause. These women also suffer a more profound drop in their testosterone levels. In considering options in replacement therapy for the premenopausal woman who has undergone hysterectomy,* the following should be considered:

The young woman who has just lost her ovaries due to surgery suffers a sudden and profound hormonal change, and is highly symptomatic and often at risk for depression—being rendered infertile is a tremendous loss.

*Actually, hysterectomy refers to removal of the uterus. Oophorectomy refers to removal of the ovaries.

These young women will generally do well on higher-dose hormone replacement, and I believe they should receive at least 1.25 mg of conjugated estrogen or the equivalent. Very often I will offer these women birth-control pills because they have a "younger" feel, and I think it is a gentler approach. I will also offer them to a young woman with premature ovarian failure—someone who didn't have a hysterectomy but whose ovaries ceased working prematurely, i.e., prior to the age of forty. In addition, estrogen levels in "the pill" are closer in strength to those of a woman's own estrogen—and, more important, taking birth-control pills is less of a daily reminder of what's different about these women. Progesterone is not needed after surgical removal of the uterus.

Testosterone

As stated in the last chapter, the ovary is not the only source of testosterone. The ovary produces only 25 percent of circulating testosterone. Other sources are the adrenal glands, the conversion by the body of other hormones into testosterone, and secretion of testosterone from the postmenopausal ovary. Thus, even though testosterone levels are lower, menopause is not necessarily associated with decreased libido.

Carefully performed research has demonstrated that testosterone supplementation enhances libido. Studies of postmenopausal women complaining of decreased libido reported a superior response to regimens containing testosterone, as compared to regimens using only estrogen. Some women also find that decreased energy levels and mood are significantly elevated with a testosterone regimen.

Testosterone use also might impair some of estrogen's beneficial, life-saving effects on cholesterol levels and heart disease.

Side effects can include increased facial-hair growth, acne, and male pattern baldness, along with permanent deepening of the voice and enlargement of the clitoris. Fortunately, with current lower-dose levels, the incidence of such side effects has decreased.

At this point, I think that testosterone should be used only in women whose decreased libido has not responded first to the use of an estrogen-containing regimen. There are two additional special circumstances where testosterone might be considered. First, following surgical menopause women may suffer a more profound drop in the circulating levels of testosterone and require replacement to support normal levels of libido and well-being. Second, patients with severe osteoporosis might be considered for testosterone supplementation. Some studies have shown that testosterone-containing regimens improve the body's response to hormone-replacement therapy.

Contraindications: Who Shouldn't Take Estrogen

Even the small number of contraindications for estrogen therapy are being re-evaluated to determine whether this treatment is harmful.

The list of contraindications is as follows:

- Unexplained vaginal bleeding
- Active liver disease and impaired liver function

- *Deep* vein blood clots—(not superficial phlebitis), with or without pulmonary emboli
- Breast cancer
- Uterine cancer, except in certain circumstances

The first three conditions are short-term problems. If and when these conditions are resolved, estrogen therapy can usually be prescribed. There is *no* question, however, that various medical situations exist—such as patients with a significantly increased risk of blood-clot formation—where the prudent practice of medicine includes a consideration of *not* prescribing estrogen. The importance of consultation between patient and physician is paramount.

The use of estrogen replacement following the successful treatment of early uterine cancer has become widespread and accepted by the medical profession. In contrast, the use of estrogen replacement for breast cancer survivors is still highly controversial and is discussed elsewhere in detail.

The Classic Side Effects

VAGINAL BLEEDING

Given a choice, most women would prefer to avoid withdrawal bleeding. When successful, taking estrogen via the continuous regimen will result in no vaginal bleeding after the initial first year. However, getting through that first year is often troublesome. Indeed, in the first two years after menopause, patients are less likely to respond favorably to continuous treatment and may need cyclic treatment to allow periodic shedding of the uterine lining.

Adjustments of medication—both in dosage *and* type of hormones—may be required, but most often the problem is eventually resolved. If bleeding problems persist, there may be a need to investigate whether there are any fibroids or polyps that might require treatment.

BLOATING AND BREAST TENDERNESS

When due to *estrogen*, these symptoms may be relieved by lowering the dose or changing the type of estrogen administered. Changing to a cyclic regimen or discontinuing estrogen for a few days may also be advantageous. Occasionally a diuretic may be used successfully.

Though scientific data are lacking, it seems clinically evident that there is a group of patients who do not tolerate progesterone administration well, complaining of bloating and breast tenderness, often accompanied by depressive mood change. Decreasing the dose or changing the type of progesterone might be effective. In addition, consideration should be given to using one of the newer, every-two-month or every-three-month regimens.

In cases where even a dose adjustment does not seem to alleviate the symptoms, it is conceivable that one may use unopposed estrogen. However, in this worst-case scenario, the price to be paid would be a yearly endometrial biopsy, or perhaps a sonogram, to make sure that no abnormal cells are developing.

WEIGHT GAIN

I am listing this as a side effect only because everybody is worried about it. But it's not true.*

*For further discussion, see pages 105–106.

Concluding Thoughts

Regarding the various hormonal regimens, the basic take-home lessons are:

- Oral estrogen is clearly better than "the patch." Transdermal estrogen does not significantly increase cardioprotective HDL. It should be used only if all else fails, or under special circumstances such as elevated triglyceride levels.
- The choice of progesterone should be limited to either Provera or pure micronized progesterone. Provera has been widely used for years. Though not all studies agree, the metabolic effects of Provera and micronized progesterone appear to be similar. We await the results of further research.

All the concern about estrogen is *not* about side effects. Multiple studies confirm that the great majority of women feel better on estrogen replacement. It's about perception. If a *need* for treatment is perceived and accepted by a patient, any side effects will surely be better tolerated.

Of prime importance is that women choose hormone replacement—*any* regimen, at *any* reasonable replacement dose needed to feel well and live longer.

8

"DESIGNER" ESTROGENS:
Scandalous Follies of the Nineties

If "Scandalous Follies" was the name of a Gilbert and Sullivan light opera, it might be mildly amusing. But it's not. Rather, in my view, it represents the worst aspects of our modern-day medical-pharmaceutical complex, aided and abetted by a sound-bite culture all too willing to digest anything the media and Madison Avenue dish out as "information."

There are so many things wrong, and my anger about the issues is so profound, that, frankly, I barely know where to begin.

The story starts with tamoxifen, the first "designer" estrogen. It seems that tamoxifen acts like estrogen on some tissues, such as the uterus and vagina, but is an "anti-estrogen" on breast tissue. And, lo and behold, it turns out to be an excellent treatment for breast cancer patients—reducing cancer recurrence in the opposite breast by about one-half. It also improves short-term mortality by 15 to 20 percent, and improves five-year survival rate by about 25 percent. It is recommended for use for up to five years. I certainly have no quarrel with the careful use of tamoxifen in appropriate, selected patients with breast cancer. I do, however, have serious concerns regarding its potential use as an alternative hormone-replacement therapy for most women.

The problem is that tamoxifen causes uterine cancer—at a rate of 2.5 to 7.5 times higher than in women who don't take tamoxifen. This increased risk was reported by the National Surgical Breast and Bowel Project (NSABP) B-14 Study, a study designed to determine the effectiveness of tamoxifen as a breast cancer treatment. After a critical review of their own data, these researchers stated that tamoxifen was guilty "only" of increasing uterine cancer risk two and a half times. Nonetheless, that tamoxifen causes substantially higher rates of uterine cancer is beyond dispute. So on to the next bad thing about tamoxifen.

The uterine cancers that tamoxifen causes are more *aggressive* and *deadly* than those that occur in women not taking tamoxifen. In a study by Magriples, using the Yale Tumor Registry, the investigators found that 67 percent of the tamoxifen-treated patients had high-grade ("bad") tumors, as compared with 24 percent in the untreated group. The outlook for patients with high-grade tumors is, of course, much worse than for those patients with low-grade tumors.

Yet another bad thing about tamoxifen is that it causes a two- to fourfold increase in blood clots, including serious deep-vein phlebitis and pulmonary emboli. Tamoxifen is not as good for your heart and blood vessels as is estrogen. You still get hot flashes, and you can include an increased incidence of cataracts and other eye damage for good measure.

Certainly if you have breast cancer and you are an appropriate candidate for tamoxifen, you still come out ahead by taking it—especially when modern techniques for monitoring the uterus are used. But, flushed with success from treatment of breast cancer, and fully aware of the desperate populace wanting to *prevent* this disease, some researchers decided to give it to healthy women.

There were warnings about this as early as 1985. Killacky reported endometrial cancer occurring in three patients on tamoxifen, and approximately one hundred other cases were described in a series of twenty-five reports. Commenting on this information, Dr. Bernard Fisher, director of the NSABP cancer studies, somewhat dryly stated that "the heterogeneity of the information in most of these reports precludes attaching much significance to the findings, other than to acknowledge that [uterine] tumors have occurred in tamoxifen-treated breast cancer patients." It was under this blind banner of "not attaching much significance," in a landscape cluttered with billboard warning signs, that the National Cancer Institute undertook its own Breast Cancer Prevention Trial. Our government and our medical research community gave tamoxifen to half of 13,388 women *without* invasive breast cancer.

The study was stopped by the researchers after four years—one year ahead of schedule. Here are the results, based upon a *press release* (not published in a medical journal).

- The incidence of breast cancer was 45 percent lower with tamoxifen use. Breast cancer occurred in 85 women on tamoxifen versus 154 on placebo.

- There were fewer osteoporotic fractures in women taking tamoxifen.

That's the end of the "good news."

Tamoxifen also caused:

- Increased uterine cancer (33 versus 14)
- Increased pulmonary emboli (17 versus 6)
- Increased major venous thrombi (30 versus 19)

There were *no* beneficial effects on heart disease.

It gets worse. Even the "good news" doesn't hold up. Two studies recently published in the medical journal *Lancet* found absolutely *no* reduction in breast cancer with tamoxifen use. Trevor Powles of Oxford, England, reported on 2,471 women followed for six years on average; Umberto Veronesi, a highly prominent breast-cancer researcher from Italy, reported on 5,408 women followed for four years on average. In the Italian study, 54 women experienced thrombophlebitis or emboli, 38 of whom were on tamoxifen, versus only 18 taking placebo.

As stated in the *Lancet* editorial, "The failure of these trials to confirm the result of the U.S. study, however, casts doubts on the wisdom of the rush, at least in some places, to prescribe tamoxifen widely for prevention."

The editors did go on to say that maybe the European studies included younger patients and perhaps patients with different risk factors than those in the U.S. study. In my view, however, this hope is thoroughly undermined by the fact that, in the NSABP B-14 Study, continued tamoxifen use after five years actually *decreased* survival rates.

After five years of tamoxifen use, breast cancer patients were then randomly selected either to continue on tamoxifen or stop it (take a placebo). Four years later, the following was apparent:

Survival (92 percent versus 86 percent) and metastases-free survival (96 percent versus 90 percent) was *better* in those patients who *stopped* tamoxifen.

As stated by Umberto Veronesi, "These data could be interpreted as being compatible with the hypothesis that long-term tamoxifen therapy is associated with a more aggressive form of breast cancer recurrence." In other words, tamoxifen, or tamoxifen-like drugs, might *appear* to prevent breast cancer, but *perhaps the only thing being accomplished is a temporary delay in the growth of small, hidden tumors. Ultimately, after several years, a more aggressive tumor might surface and be more difficult to treat.*

So perhaps our U.S. scientists were premature in halting the tamoxifen study after only four years. Perhaps any "protective effect" would disappear after long-term use. Frankly, what this suggests to me is that both the beginning *and* the end of the National Cancer Institute Study were suspect.

Personally, I would never have conducted the tamoxifen research that was foisted upon an unknowing, trusting, and (as far as breast cancer prevention is concerned) desperate public. The scientists may have realized that serious uterine cancer was occurring early in the study. When the scientists finally stopped the study one year early (the party line being that tamoxifen had proven so effective in preventing breast cancer that there was no point in continuing it) I wonder whether they were also trying to prevent any further deadly harm from uterine cancers caused by tamoxifen.

By the way, did you catch the "luncheon" given by

these researchers, ostensibly for the patients who were part of their study? As I mentioned, it was necessary to circulate a press release about the findings because the researchers hadn't yet published them. Other doctors and researchers had *not* been able to examine the data. Nonetheless, this "tamoxifen tea party" was given great fanfare, complete with happily televised researchers disingenuously suggesting "caution" in interpreting their results. Given how fast they were to start the study despite early warning signs of danger, how determined they were to continue it despite the appearance of rather significant side effects, and how eager they were to then jump in front of a TV camera, "cautious" is not a word that immediately comes to mind.

Enter Evista

In yet another breach of prudent judgment, our government bestowed an additional "gift" to women's *and* men's health care recently—by allowing prescription drugs to be marketed directly to patients. The "selling" of Evista is a prime example.

Did you know: There's life after menopause. Actually, I may not be able to say that. Let me try again. *"There's life after menopause," TRADEMARK.* Yes, Virginia, it's true: The catchphrase "life after menopause" is now the sole trademark property of the drug company that manufactures raloxifene (Evista).

Raloxifene is the newest "designer" estrogen. It is chemically related to tamoxifen. In an article entitled "Behind the Buzz on Designer Estrogens, Questions Linger," the *New York Times* accurately calls it a "cousin" of tamoxifen. (Both are SERMs.)* But in the same article, the *Times* writer also states that "There are drawbacks with estrogen. . . . It presents a three to five times greater-than-normal risk of uterine cancer." This is profoundly misleading and inaccurate—all too typical of the deteriorating accuracy and trustworthiness of personal-health journalism. And this article was actually one of the best I've seen.

The buzz about "designer" estrogens infuriates me. There is no question that it would be great to modulate and select the estrogen receptors of various tissues, turning some on (heart, brain, and bone) and others off (breast and uterus). Fantasy is always great.

I first heard this buzz in my office from my patients, who told me that there was a "new estrogen" that "prevented breast cancer." This was fully one year before I saw *anything* resembling a published medical journal article about it. In fact, at that time, there was more information available about Evista in my stockbroker's research report about the drug company.

The buzz is that raloxifene *decreases* breast cancer in the *first 30 months of use.* Well now, haven't we heard *that* before?

In case you missed it, in the introduction I referred to raloxifene/Evista as a third-rate, flash-in-the-pan substitute for estrogen. Here's why:

- Evista does *not* increase HDL ("good") cholesterol, and almost certainly will *not* provide as much protection against heart disease as estrogen does.

*The acronym SERM stands for Selective Estrogen Receptor Modulator. These are molecules that stimulate only certain estrogen receptors. In theory, SERMs would effect only those tissues necessary to obtain desired benefits, while not effecting those tissues which could increase risk.

- Evista does *not* lower LDL ("bad") cholesterol to the extent that estrogen does. There is a reduction of between 8 and 11 percent using raloxifene versus 15 to 20 percent using estrogen.
- Evista has *no* effect on hot flashes.
- Evista almost certainly will have *no* effect on Alzheimer's disease—a disease that affects 40 percent of women over eighty. Estrogen use stands to save millions of lives by preventing perhaps 30 to 60 percent of Alzheimer's disease cases. Evista forsakes these millions of lives.
- Evista doesn't improve cognitive function. Estrogen does.
- Depending upon which study you believe, Evista may be more harmful or the same as estrogen regarding blood clots.
- Evista is even mediocre regarding osteoporosis, the "prevention"—*not* treatment—of which is the only thing the FDA approved it for. Bone turnover is decreased 50 percent by estrogen and only 30 percent by Evista. One researcher has said that in this regard Evista is like "half-strength estrogen."

Let me give the devil his due. First, Evista does cause much less stimulation of uterine and breast tissues. The uterine lining stays quite thin and quiescent on Evista. (Mind you, since tamoxifen—the "cousin" of raloxifene—causes increased uterine cancer, you can be sure that the drug company that manufactures raloxifene made absolutely sure that its product caused no such problem with uterine cancer.) Second, women taking Evista have much less breast tenderness, reflecting its probable decreased stimulation of breast tissue.

But I still have trouble with a potential *third* advantage of Evista—a decreased incidence of breast cancer. Even if early studies on raloxifene show a decreased incidence of breast cancer, the following should be kept in mind about its close relative:

- The tamoxifen study in the United States was refuted by two other studies.
- Long-term use of tamoxifen might actually be counterproductive and dangerous. Early cancer growth might be delayed, only to appear later as more aggressive tumors. (Presumably raloxifene use could follow the same pattern.)
- Heart disease is still far and away the number-one killer of postmenopausal women. In this regard, raloxifene offers precious few of estrogen's life-saving benefits.

When it comes to choosing hormone treatments, it's all about heart disease and blood-vessel disease. Second to that, it's all about brain function and Alzheimer's. Compared to estrogen, Evista is at best second-rate regarding heart disease and absolutely ineffective regarding the brain and Alzheimer's disease. Hence, *third rate*.

Drug companies are already working on the next generation of "designer" estrogens. I'm sure they will leave Evista users twisting slowly in the wind as they move on to different drugs and greener pastures. By contrast, estrogen has been in use for half a century. Hence, *flash in the pan*.

All of which brings me to the closing act of "Scandalous Follies of the Nineties."

The "Selling" of Designer Estrogens: Let the Buyer Beware

With all the "drug money" (pharmaceutical research funding) around, there are more professors working for more pharmaceutical companies than ever before. Frankly, I don't know how it's possible to give an intellectually honest lecture about a drug like Evista when a company representative is sitting in the audience *and* they're paying the speaker. In a recent, hour-long lecture, one such professor-salesman conveniently left out any mention of Alzheimer's disease, the risk of which is significantly reduced by estrogen but *not* by Evista. This kind of intellectual dishonesty by otherwise brilliant people greatly disturbs me.

A published ad for Evista has all the straightforwardness of a car-lease advertisement—legal, but close to the line. Frankly, I don't much care about car-lease ads. I *expect* to pay $2,500 up front despite the mention of "no money down." I *don't* expect—nor should any of us tolerate—even a *hint* of the written sleight-of-hand about an issue upon which millions of lives depend.

In my opinion, for the FDA (or whichever "responsible" agency) to have allowed drug companies to advertise prescription drugs directly to the public is unconscionable.

In this age of capitalism, some might say you can't blame drug companies for a bit of old-fashioned advertising. I beg to differ. Evista was approved only for the *prevention* of osteoporosis—*not* its *treatment,* much less anything else. Yet the advertisements talk about estrogen, cholesterol, breast cancer, and uterine cancer with a car-lease-ad regard for the truth. And of course, it ends with "There's life after menopause." *Trademark.*

Well, there's heart disease after menopause. There's Alzheimer's disease after menopause. There are hot flashes and mood changes and cognitive function deterioration after menopause. There's even osteoporosis after menopause, for which Evista is second rate. Estrogen will save millions of lives and improve millions more—Evista won't. Its potential reduction of breast-cancer growth *pales* in comparison to the profound benefits it *won't* provide.

Compared to estrogen, which has been studied for half a century, these newer synthetic hormones are in their infancy. Though the *theory* of selecting beneficial effects while avoiding possible harmful effects is of course attractive, the ideal compound has not yet been found. Hopefully, future research will lead to its discovery and implementation. Until then, the widespread use of any designer estrogen would be premature.

9

CONCLUDING THOUGHTS

Estrogen saves lives.

That estrogen can prevent the premature deaths of tens of thousands of women each year in the United States alone is both astonishing *and* tragic. For some time I have felt personally and professionally burdened by what I view as an almost genocidal underuse of estrogen, a hormone whose natural capabilities confer an extraordinary survival advantage upon women. By choosing not to replace estrogen after it has been lost, the all-too-large majority of menopausal women worldwide refuse one of nature's gifts.

Though my credentials include years of clinical practice, teaching, and study of obstetrics and gynecology, I am *not* one of the highly published professors from whose brilliant work I liberally quote and continue to learn. Nonetheless, this is my good-faith effort to "move the stone"—to beg your consideration of hormone replacement in the light of our ever-growing knowledge. I have endeavored to provide a foundation of such knowledge (albeit accompanied occasionally by passionate editorial) to more fully enable a woman's informed choice regarding this most profound issue.

Women must recognize the preeminent role of heart disease and blood-vessel disease, and the extraordinary impact of estrogen on the cardiovascular system. *One or two million* more women in the United States can reach the age of seventy-five in the first part of the next century if estrogen use increases. Currently, these lives are being lost prematurely.

One million women each year in the United States suffer from bone fractures largely due to osteoporosis. The resulting level of disability and death is staggering. Estrogen is no less remarkable in its ability to prevent the greater portion of this malady, preserving quality of life and extending lives in large number.

Estrogen's effects on the anatomy, function, and health of brain cells are astonishing. If estrogen can indeed prevent 30 to 60 percent of Alzheimer's disease—*which itself affects 40 percent of women over the age of eighty*—millions more lives will be extended and saved.

If women can be convinced that breast cancer is only minimally, *if at all*, related to estrogen therapy—and that even a worst-case scenario results in a loss of life that is but a small fraction of lives saved by proven benefits—perhaps a significant barrier to estrogen use will be removed.

As continued research and education lends credence to the advantages of hormone replacement, perhaps more women will perceive a *need* for estrogen and better tolerate any side effects. As regards hormone replacement, fully one-half of women *don't even fill their prescriptions* and less than one-quarter continue estrogen for even a few years.

The dissemination of accurate, credible information is therefore of vital importance. In this regard, we must "raise the level of our game" and retreat from our simplistic sound-bite approach. Tabloid journalism has no place in the health care of women and men.

As witness their increasing use of exaggerated statistical terminology, such as *relative risk*, even our formerly staid medical journals are not immune to the forces of our culture. With less emphasis being placed on the bottom line, *absolute risk*, it has become increasingly difficult for both doctor and patient to gauge the importance of newly reported medical-research findings.

Furthermore, there is already enough confusion without the direct marketing of prescription drugs to patients. This particular FDA folly should immediately cease and desist. The pharmaceutical industry cannot be allowed to play on women's fears and distrust of hormone replacement.

I am even more concerned about any effect "consultant's fees" might have on the written and spoken words of our most brilliant scientific talent. The future of women's health depends on their integrity.

The medical-research community should also think twice about conducting studies where women *are randomly assigned* to take either estrogen or placebo pills for years on end. In view of our evolving knowledge regarding the profound effects of estrogen on a woman's health and life, that her choice should be relegated to the "flip of a coin" is at best ethically questionable—if not a reprehensible and retrogressive lapse.

But enough of that. This book is about life. It is only in the twentieth century that life expectancy passed the age of fifty, beginning the modern era of life after menopause.

This modern era of happily prolonged life has been a product of our adaptability, our intellect, and our hearts. The scientific achievements which have improved the health of mankind are as natural as life itself. With estrogen, nature bestows a gift of improved health and prolonged life upon women. Our evolving insight and knowledge of our bodies is yet another gift.

We should carefully, and gratefully, partake of the wonders of these gifts.

APPENDIX A

SAVING LIVES WITH ESTROGEN:

A Look at the Numbers

In the introduction, I discussed the work of Dr. Robin Gorsky, which predicted 6 *percent* more women surviving to age seventy-five if they took estrogen from the beginning of their menopause at age fifty. I also stated that, because this involved *tens of millions* of menopausal women in the United States, that *tens of thousands* of lives each year could be saved by increased estrogen use.

I will now provide you with a summary of two additional studies and U.S. population data for your consideration. You can use the information provided to make your own calculations and critical observations. All in all, I think you'll find the predicted number of lives saved both accurate and thought-provoking.

The Population Data

THE OLDER U.S. FEMALE POPULATION

Age	1990		2000		2010		2020	
55–64	10.8 million	(8.6%)	12.1 million	(9.0%)	17.1 million	(12.1%)	19.3 million	(12.9%)
65–74	10.1	(8.1%)	9.8	(7.3%)	11.0	(7.8%)	15.6	(10.4%)
>75	7.8	(6.2%)	9.3	(7.0%)	9.8	(6.9%)	11.0	(7.3%)
Total	28.7		31.2		37.9		45.9	

Data from U.S. Bureau of the Census, "Projections of the Population of the United States: 1977–2050" *Current Population Reports*, Series P-25, No. 704.

These figures support my assertion that there will be 35 million women aged fifty to seventy-five early in the next century (mentioned in discussion of the Gorsky study), and 10 to 15 million women aged sixty-five to seventy-four during that time frame (referred to in the following study by Dr. Lobo).

Calculations of Lives Saved: The Lobo Study

In 1995, Dr. Rogerio Lobo, chairman of Ob-Gyn at Columbia University College of Physicians and Surgeons, published an article in *The American Journal of Obstetrics and Gynecology* entitled, "Benefits and Risks of Estrogen Replacement." Dr. Lobo calculated estimates of *annual* lives saved by estrogen-replacement therapy (ERT) per 100,000 women aged sixty-five to seventy-four, again based on the *presumed* benefits and risks of taking estrogen.

As can be seen on the next page, 366 lives per 100,000 population are saved each year versus at most 38 lives lost to breast cancer.* Dr. Lobo also included 26 lives lost to uterine cancer, which is almost certainly no longer true. For the sake of argument, let's agree on an even 300 lives

*Modified from Dr. Rogerio Lobo

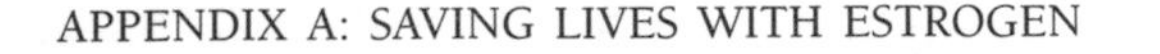

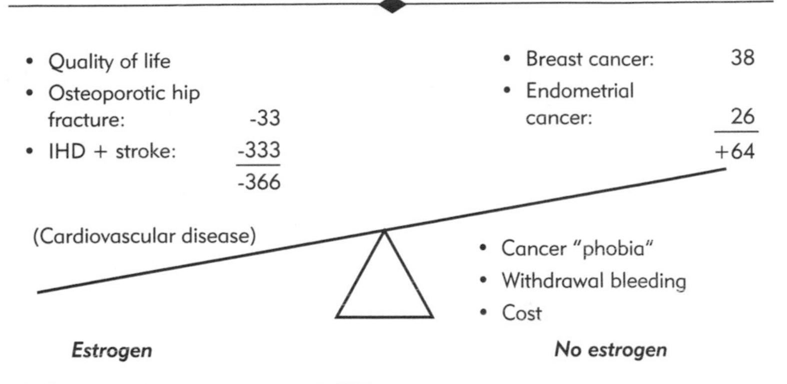

* Conjugated equine estrogens 0.825

Risk versus benefit of ERT, calculated as a change in mortality annually per 100,000 women aged 65 to 74, shows that mortality is improved with estrogen use. On the positive side, lives saved because of reductions in osteoporotic hip fractures and in ischemic heart disease *(IHD)* and stroke number 33 and 333, respectively. On negative side, two major risk factors related to estrogen use, breast cancer and endometrial cancer, result in 38 and 26 lives lost, respectively, with estrogen use, or a total of 64 lives lost per year per 100,000 women.

Data from R. Lobo, "Benefits and Risks of Estrogen Replacement Therapy," *The American Journal of Obstetrics and Gynecology* 173:982, 1995.

saved per 100,000 women each year. It is important to consider the following:

> In the year 2000 there will be *10 million* women aged sixty-five to seventy-four.
>
> In the year 2020 there will be *15 million* women aged sixty-five to seventy-four.
>
> **300** lives saved per 100,000 women each year equals
>
> *30,000 lives saved* per 10 million women each year (as of the year 2000), and
>
> *45,000 lives saved* per 15 million women each year (as of the year 2025).

Once again, tens of thousands of lives each year in the United States are not being saved when they could be.

Because women are *not* taking estrogen, premature deaths are *not* being prevented. This loss of life is staggering. (Remember, these lives are *only* those of women *aged 65 to 74* and *only* in the U.S.)

Calculation Caveats

- *Some women are already taking estrogen:* True, but not a lot. Probably, at most, 20 percent of women are taking estrogen long-term. Noted researchers such as Henderson and Paganini-Hill have stated that the saving of lives is *twice* as great after fifteen years of estrogen use than after only seven and one-half years of estrogen use.
- *Some women shouldn't take estrogen:* True, but I certainly doubt it's more than 10 percent of the population. Presuming a most conservative approach to breast cancer—ruling out estrogen for the 2 percent of women who have had breast cancer by age 50 and the 7 percent who have it by age 70—the vast majority of the remaining 93 to 98 percent of women *can* take estrogen.
- *The degree of "benefit" is not absolutely proven:* This is true in the most scientifically narrow sense. However, not only has estrogen use been shown to reduce deaths in multiple studies, but we have discovered the how and why. *How much more information do we need?* Even if the survival benefits are *half* (3 percent) of what is likely to be true, estrogen would prevent one million rather than two million premature deaths of women in the United States over twenty-five years early in the next century.

The Henderson Study

This study looked at women taking Premarin from age fifty to age seventy-five, and the cumulative lives saved per 100,000 women. It was mentioned in the above article by Dr. Lobo, but the original work was published in 1986—something that I find both startling and disquieting.

CHANGE IN MORTALITY WITH ORAL ERT*

Condition	*Relative risk*	*Cumulative change/100,000*
Osteoporotic fractures	0.4	−563
Gallbladder disease	1.5	+2
Endometrial cancer	2.0	+63†
Breast cancer	1.1	+187
Ischemic heart disease	0.5	−5250
Net change		**−5561**
Net % change		−41

Modified from D. D. Henderson, et al. *The American Journal of Obstetrics and Gynecology* 1986: 154: 1181–6.
*Conjugated equine estrogens 0.625 mg/day in women aged 50 to 75 years.
†Case rate: 0.05.
From R. Lobo, Benefits and Risks of Estrogen Replacement Therapy, 173:982, 1995.

I draw your attention to the *net change* of 5,561 lives saved out of 100,000 women aged 50 to 75.

5,561 per 100,000 =
55 per 1000 =
5.5 per 100 =
5.5%

This is a 5.5% survival advantage accruing to menopausal women taking estrogen from ages fifty to seventy-five. That the calculations of Gorsky, Lobo, and Henderson are so consistent is really quite remarkable. That they have been languishing, unnoticed, since as early as 1986, is tragic.

Feel free to incorporate any numbers you choose. It is my considered opinion that estrogen confers a 6 percent survival advantage (certainly no less than 3 percent) to menopausal women. This figure does not even consider any additional benefits from the reduction of Alzheimer's disease—which is likely to be extremely important. Worst-case scenarios of lives lost to breast cancer are *overwhelmed* by these profound, life-saving benefits.

Lest I be accused of exaggeration, may I point out that tens of thousands of lives lost annually refers *only* to menopausal women in the United States. After all, we all live on the same planet. So we may actually have to *multiply* the number of lives saved by a factor of 10 or 20 if we consider that the tragic underuse of estrogen is truly worldwide.

APPENDIX B

TRUTH, LIES, AND STATISTICS:
Understanding Relative and Absolute Risk

We have become a culture inundated by "sound bites." How often have we heard that eating a particular (and usually delicious) food increases our risk of heart attack by *20 percent*? Such warnings have all the earmarks of your basic late-twentieth-century sound bite. Armed with such dramatic statistics, professors, researchers, and epidemiologists feel empowered to emerge from their otherwise invisible professional lives for a well-earned bit of TV fame (after all, 20 percent is important, isn't it?). The medical journals, also, are all too happy to be quoted in the media. These journals also seem to have subtly changed their editorial policies to present scientific evidence in as statistically dramatic a fashion as possible.

Finally, this well-orchestrated hoopla is integrated into our culture by America's very own Madison Avenue. We need only buy foodstuffs identified by that life-preserving (reduced fat) green triangle on the package, and our immortality is assured.

What the public is *not* told, taught, or even asked to consider, is that 20 percent may only turn out to be the difference between a 1 in a thousand risk of a heart attack that year and a 1.2 in a thousand risk. Viewed this way, the particular degree of increased risk (20 percent) doesn't seem so daunting. *Now* it may not be "late-breaking news," and *now* the various health professionals and publications may have to remain in relative obscurity. We might even be tempted to stare danger in the face and purchase a buttery French pastry without any of those green labels.

Doctors and patients alike are being inundated daily with information about *relative* risk. If a study shows that the risk changes from a 1 in X chance to a 1.2 in X chance, it is *always* true that the *relative* risk had increased 20 percent—no argument from me. *But*, when it's time to make important decisions about our health and our lives, it seems to me vitally important that we know the *absolute* risk involved. This way, we can all understand the magnitude of what's being discussed and can make our *own* informed value judgments about how important some statistical finding is.

So let me attempt to add a realistic and accurate perspective to some commonly discussed *absolute* risks. Let's try to develop a mental picture of 1 in 10,000 and 1 in 100,000, using *inches* as a basic measurement.

10,000 inches = 833 feet
833 feet = approximately the height of an 80- or 90-story building
It seems fair to say that an 80- or 90-story building = a *skyscraper.*

Therefore,

1 in 10,000 = 1 inch in a *skyscraper.*

Similarly,

100,000 inches = 8,333 feet
8,333 feet = about 1½ miles (for simplicity's sake, let's call it a mile)

Therefore,

1 in 100,000 = 1 inch in a *mile.*

Armed with this new perspective, let's look at a hypothetical situation where the *relative risk* is *doubled* from 2 to 4.

When risk changes from 2 in 100 to 4 in 100 (that is, from 2 *percent* to 4 *percent*) it certainly seems worthy of serious consideration.

A change from 2 in 1,000 to 4 in 1,000 = 0.2 versus 0.4 percent, or 1 in 500 versus 1 in 250.

This level of risk gives everybody trouble. For example, physicians and mothers-to-be often decide about whether to perform an amniocentesis based on such numbers. We just have to reflect as best we can and follow the dictates of our hearts and minds. However, this level of risk can be especially important when talking about huge numbers (e.g., millions of women taking estrogen).

Consider: 2 in 10,000 versus 4 in 10,000 = two inches versus four inches of risk *along the length of a skyscraper.* The media and medical profession love to tell us about the *doubled* risk. They never emphasize the skyscraper.

Consider also: 2 in 100,000 versus 4 in 100,000 = two inches versus four inches out of a mile. In this case, it's the same "doubled" risk, but an extra few inches out of a whole mile doesn't exactly make me panic. In fact, I'm always amazed that scientists can discover such a small effect.

Thus the moral of the story is that patients and doctors alike should *never* consider the importance of *relative risk* without immediately being told about *absolute risk.* If you don't know the absolute risk, then you don't know how to consider the importance of the finding. Medical education should not be predicated on some "doubled" or "tripled" risk, which becomes the fodder for hype and distortion. We should be told whether the risk involves extra percentage points or just a couple of inches out of a skyscraper, or a mile.

This may not make for hard-hitting TV news. In fact, serious medical information is often quite tedious, somewhat dull, and often conflicted for years. We need to learn together in an environment uncluttered by vanity and hype. Our very lives depend upon the growth of accurate medical knowledge.

BIBLIOGRAPHY

SUGGESTED MEDICAL REFERENCES

Special mention should be made of the writings of Leon Speroff, M.D. (coauthors Robert H. Glass, M.D., and Nathan G. Kase, M.D.), whose texts regarding the complex interplay between women's hormones have set the standard for thoughtful analysis and insight for generations of physicians. Transcripts of his discussions with leading investigators regarding the strengths and weaknesses of estrogen in relation to breast cancer and heart disease are particularly noteworthy.

The teaching materials, journals, and research meetings of the North American Menopause Society (Cleveland, Ohio) are also quite remarkable.

A Clinical Guide for the Care of Older Women. Primary and Preventive Care, second edition, Bygny RL, Speroff L. Williams & Wilkins, 1996.

Clinical Gynecologic Endocrinology and Infertility, fifth edition, Speroff L, Glass RH, Kase NG. Williams Wilkins, 1994.

Speroff L. Postmenopausal hormone therapy and breast cancer. Oregon Health Sciences University School of Medicine, 1997. *Contemporary Ob/Gyn,* Vol. 42, No. 1 (Suppl).

Speroff L. Postmenopausal hormone therapy and cardiovascular system. Oregon Health Sciences University School of Medicine, 1997. *Contemporary Ob/Gyn,* Vol. 42, No. 6 (Suppl).

Treatment of the Postmenopausal Woman. Basic and Clinical Aspects. Lobo RA (editor). Raven Press, NY, 1994.

INTRODUCTION

Andrews WC. Menopause and hormone replacement: Introduction. *Obstetrics Gynecology* 87:15, 1996.

Bachmann GA, Simon JA, Sorrel PM. Considerations in managing your HRT patients. *Contemporary Obstetrics and Gynecology* 34, 1997.

Barrett-Connor E. Risks and benefits of replacement estrogen. *Annual Review of Medicine* 43:239, 1992.

Brinton LA, Schairer C. Postmenopausal hormone-replacement therapy—time for a reappraisal? *New England Journal of Medicine* 336:1821, 1997.

Campbell S, Whitehead M. Estrogen therapy and the menopausal syndrome. *Clinical Obstetrics and Gynecology* 4:31, 1997.

Criqui MH, Suarez L, Barrett-Connor E, et al. Postmenopausal estrogen use and mortality. *American Journal of Epidemiology* 128:606, 1998.

Ettinger B, Friedman GD, Bush T, Quesenberrh CP. Reduced mortality associated with long-term postmenopausal estrogen therapy. *Obstetrics Gynecology* 87:6, 1996.

Fries JF. Aging, illness and health policy: Implications of the compression of morbidity. *Perspectives in Biological Medicine* 31:407, 1988.

Fries JF, Green LW, Levine S. Health promotion and the compression of morbidity. *Lancet* 1:481, 1989.

Gerhard M, Ganz P. How do we explain the clinical benefits of estrogen? *Circulation* 92:5, 1995.

Gorsky RD, Koplan JP, Peterson HB, Thacker SB. Relative risks and benefits of long-term estrogen replacement therapy: a decision analysis. *Obstetrics Gynecology* 83:161, 1994.

Grady D, Rubin SM, Petitti DB, et al. Hormone therapy to prevent disease and prolong life in postmenopausal women. *Annals of Internal Medicine* 117:1016, 1992.

Grodstein F, Stampfer MJ, Colditz GA. Postmenopausal hormone therapy and mortality. *New England Journal of Medicine* 336:1769, 1997.

Hammond CB. Menopause and hormone replacement therapy: an overview. *Obstetrics Gynecology* 87:2S, 1996.

Hammond CB, Jelovsek FR, Lee KL, et al. Effects of long-term estrogen replacement therapy: I. Metabolic effects. *American Journal of Obstetrics and Gynecology* 133:525, 1979.

Henderson AE, Paganini-Hill A, Ross RK. Decreased mortality in users of estrogen replacement therapy. *Archives of Internal Medicine* 151:76, 1991.

Lobo R, Pickar JH, Wild RA, Walsh B, Hirvonen E, for The Menopause Study Group. Metabolic impact of adding medroxyprogesterone acetate to conjugated estrogen therapy in postmenopausal women. *In press.*

Newman KP, Sullivan JM. Coronary heart disease in women: epidemiology clinical syndromes, and management. *Journal of the North American Menopause Society* 3:51, 1996.

The North American Menopause Society. Achieving long-term continuance of menopausal ERT/HRT: consensus opinion of the North American Menopause Society. *Journal of the North American Menopause Society* 5:69, 1998.

Petitti DB, Perlman JA, Sidney S. Noncontraceptive estrogens and mortality: long-term follow-up of women in the Walnut Creek Study. *Obstetrics Gynecology* 70:289, 1987.

Salamone LM, Pressman AR, Seeley DG, Cauley JA. Estrogen replacement therapy: a survey of older women's attitudes. *Archives of Internal Medicine* 156:1293, 1996.

Schwartz PE. Hormone replacement therapy after cancers of the reproductive tract. North American Menopause Society, 8th annual meeting, 1997.

Thompson W. Estrogen replacement therapy in practice: trends and issues. *The American Journal of Obstetrics and Gynecology* 173:990, 1995.

Utian WH. Menopause: a modern perspective from a controversial history. *Progress in the Management of the Menopause* 1, 1997.

CHAPTER 1
DECREASING THE FEAR OF BREAST CANCER: A FIRST STEP

Armstrong BK. Oestrogen therapy after the menopause—boon or bone? *Medical Journal of Australia* 148:213–214, 1988.

Bergkvist L, Adami H O, Persson I, et al. The risk of breast cancer after estrogen and estrogen-progestin replacement. *New England Journal of Medicine* 321:293–297, 1989.

Bergkvist L, Adami H-O, Persson I, et al. Prognosis after breast cancer diagnosis in women exposed to estrogen and estrogen-progestogen replacement therapy. *American Journal of Epidemiology* 130:221–227, 1989.

Bonnier P, Romain S, Giacolone L, et al. Clinical and biologic prognostic factors in breast cancer diagnosed during postmenopausal hormone replacement therapy. *Obstetrics Gynecology* 85:11, 1997.

Brewster WR, DiSaia PJ. Estrogen replacement therapy in breast cancer survivors. North American Menopause Society, 8th annual meeting, 1997.

Brinton LA, Hoover R, Fraumeni JF Jr. Menopausal oestrogens and breast cancer risk: an expanded case-control study. *British Journal of Cancer* 54:825, 1986.

Colditz GA, Egan KM, Stampfer MJ. Hormone replacement therapy and risk of breast cancer: results from epidemiologic studies. *American Journal of Obstetrics and Gynecology* 168:1473–80, 1993.

Colditz GA, Hankinson SE, Hunter DJ, et al. Use of estrogens and progestins and the risk of breast cancer in postmenopausal women. *New England Journal of Medicine* 332:1589–93, 1995.

Colditz GA, Stampfer MJ, Willett WC, et al. Type of postmenopausal hormone use and risk of breast cancer: 12-year follow-up from the Nurses Health Study. *Cancer Causes Control* 3:433–439, 1992.

Couzi RJ, Kilzlsover KJ, Fetting JH. Prevalence of menopausal symptoms among women with a history of breast cancer and attitudes toward estrogen replacement therapy. *Journal of Clinical Oncology* 13:2737, 1995.

DeMott K. HRT use may increase risk for breast cancer. *Obstretic/Gynecologic News* 6, Jan 1998.

DiSaia PJ, Grosen EA, Kurosaki T, et al. Hormone replacement therapy in breast cancer survivors: a cohort study. *Obstetrics Gynecology* 174:1495, 1996.

Dupont WD, Page DL. Menopausal estrogen replacement therapy and breast cancer. *Archives of Internal Medicine* 151:67–72, 1991.

Dupont WD, Page DL, Rogers LW, Parl FF. Influence of exogenous estrogens, proliferative breast disease, and other variables on breast cancer risk. *Cancer* 63:948–57, 1989.

Ellison PT, O'Rourke MT. Age and prognosis in premenopausal breast cancer. *Lancet* 342:60, 1993.

Gambrell RD Jr., Babgnell CA, Greenblatt RB. Role of estrogens and progesterone in the etiology and prevention of endometrial cancer: a review. *The American Journal of Obstetrics and Gynecology* 146:696, 1983.

Gambrell RD Jr., Maier RC, Sanders BI. Decreased incidence of breast cancer in postmenopausal estrogen-progestogen users. *Obstetrics Gynecology* 62:435–43, 1983.

Gammon MD, Thompson WD. Infertility and breast cancer: a population-based case-control study. *American Journal of Epidemiology* 132:708, 1990.

Gammon MD, Thompson WD. Polycystic ovaries and the risk of breast cancer. *American Journal of Epidemiology* 134:818, 1991.

Guinee VF, Olsson H, Moller T, et al. Effect of pregnancy on prognosis for young women with breast cancer. *Lancet* 343:1587–1589, 1994.

Henderson BE, Paganini-Hill A, Ross RK. Decreased mortality in users of estrogen replacement therapy. *Archives of Internal Medicine* 151:75–78, 1991.

Hiatt RA, Bawol R, Friedman GD, Hoover R. Exogenous estrogen and breast cancer after bilateral oophorectomy. *Cancer* 54:139, 1984.

Hulka BS. Hormone-replacement therapy and the risk of breast cancer. *CA-A Cancer Journal for Clinicians* 40:289, 1990.

Kaufman DW, Palmer JR, DeMouzon J, et al. Estrogen replacement therapy and the risk of breast cancer: results from the case-control surveillance study. *American Journal of Epidemiology* 134:1375–85, 1991.

Korenman SG. The endocrinology of breast cancer. *Cancer* 46:874, 1990.

Korenman SG. Estrogen window hypothesis of the etiology of breast cancer. *Lancet* 1:700–701, 1980.

Nachtigall MJ, Smilen SW, Nachtigall RAD, Nachtigall RH, Nachtigall LI. Incidence of breast cancer in a 22-year study of women receiving estrogen-progestin replacement therapy. *Obstetrics Gynecology* 80:827, 1992.

Nugent P, O'Connell TX. Breast cancer and pregnancy. *Archives of Surgery* 120:1221, 1985.

Palmer JR, Rosenberg L, Clarke EA, Miller DR, Shapiro S. Breast cancer risk after estrogen replacement therapy: results from the Toronto Breast Cancer Study. *American Journal of Epidemiology* 134:1386–95, 1991.

Petitti DB. *Meta-analysis, decision, analysis, and cost-effectiveness analysis: methods for quantitative synthesis in medicine.* New York: Oxford University Press, 1994.

Powles TJ, Hickish T, Casey S, O'Brien M. Hormone replacement after breast cancer. *Lancet* 342:60, 1993.

Risch HA, Howe GR. Menopausal hormone usage and breast cancer in Saskatchewan: a record-linkage cohort study. *American Journal of Epidemiology* 136:670–83, 1994.

Rohan TE, McMichael AJ. Noncontraceptive exogenous oestrogen therapy and breast cancer. *Medical Journal of Australia* 148:217, 1988.

Saunders CM, Baum M. Breast cancer and pregnancy: a review. *Journal of the Royal Society of Medicine* 86:162–165, 1993.

Schairer C, Byrne C, Keyl PM, et al. Menopausal estrogen and estrogen-progestin replacement therapy and risk of breast cancer (United States). *Cancer Causes Control* 5:491–500, 1994.

Solero-Arenas M, Delgado Rodriguez M, Rodrigues-Conteras R, et al. Menopausal hormone replacement therapy and breast cancer: a meta-analysis. *Obstetrics Gynecology* 79:286–94, 1992.

Skegg DCG, Noonan EA, Paul C, et al. Depo-medroxyprogesterone acetate and breast cancer: a pooled analysis of the World Health Organization and New Zealand Studies. *Journal of the American Medical Association* 273:799–804, 1995.

Speroff L. Postmenopausal hormone therapy and breast cancer. *Obstetrics Gynecology* 87:445, 1996.

Standford JL, Weiss NS, Voight LF, et al. Combined estrogen and progestin hormone replacement therapy in relation to risk of breast cancer in middle-aged women. *Journal of the American Medical Association* 274:137–42, 1995.

Steinberg KK, Thacker SB, Smith SJ, et al. A meta-analysis of the effect of estrogen replacement therapy on the risk of breast cancer. *Journal of the American Medical Association* 265:1985–90, 1991.

Strickland DM, Gambrell RD Jr., Butzin CA, Strickland K. The relationship between breast cancer survival and prior postmenopausal estrogen use. *Obstetrics Gynecology* 80:400, 1992.

Vassilopoulou-Sellin R. Hormone replacement therapy after breast cancer diagnosis and treatment. *Menopause* 6:1, 1998.

Vassilopoulou-Sellin R, Klein MJ. Estrogen replacement therapy after treatment for localized breast carcinoma. *Cancer* 78:1043, 1996.

Voigt LF, Weiss NS, Chu JR, et al. Progestogen supplementation of exogenous oestrogens and risk of endometrial cancer. *Lancet* 338:274, 1991.

WHO collaborative study of neoplasia and steroid contraceptives. Breast cancer and depo-medroxyprogesterone acetate: a multinational study. *Lancet* 338:833–838, 1991.

Wile AG, Optell BW, Margileth DA. Hormone replacement therapy in previously treated breast cancer patients. *American Journal of Surgery* 165:372–375, 1993.

Wingo PA, Layde PM, Lee NC, Rubin G, Ory HW. The risk of breast cancer in postmenopausal women who have used estrogen replacement therapy. *Journal of the American Medical Association* 257:209, 1987.

Yang CP, Daling JR, Bond PR, et al. Noncontraceptive hormone use and risk of breast cancer. *Cancer Causes Control* 3:475, 1992.

Zemlickis D, Lishner M, Degendorter P, et al. Maternal and fetal outcome after breast cancer in pregnancy. *American Journal of Obstetrics and Gynecology* 166:781, 1992.

CHAPTER 2
SAVING LIVES: ESTROGEN AND HEART DISEASE

Adams MR, Clarkson TB, Koritnik DR. From menarche to menopause: coronary artery atherosclerosis and protection in cynomolgus monkeys. *American Journal of Obstetrics and Gynecology* 160:1280, 1989.

Adams MP, Kaplan JR, Manuck SB, et al. Inhibition of coronary artery atherosclerosis by 17-beta estradiol in ovariectomized monkeys: lack of an effect of added progesterone. *Arteriosclerosis* 10:151, 1990.

Baker ED, Castelli WP. Coronary heart disease and its risk factor among women in the Framingham Study. In Eaker ED, Packard B, Pines A, et al: The effects of hormone replacement therapy in normal postmenopausal women: measurements of Doppler-derived parameters of aortic flow. *American Journal of Obstetrics and Gynecology* 164:806, 1991.

Bar J, Tepper R, Fuchs J, et al. The effect of estrogen replacement therapy on platelet aggregation and adenosine triphosphate release in postmenopausal women. *Obstetrics Gynecology* 81:261, 1993.

Baron YM, Galea R, Brincat M. Carotid artery wall changes in estrogen-treated and untreated postmenopausal women. *Obstetrics Gynecology* 91:983, 1998.

Barrett-Connor E. Postmenopausal estrogen and prevention bias. *Annals of Internal Medicine* 115:455, 1991.

Barrett-Connor E, Wingard DL, Criqui MH. Postmenopausal estrogen use and heart disease risk factors in the 1980s. *Journal of the American Medical Association* 261:2095, 1989.

Beard CM, Kotte TE, Annegers JF, Ballard DJ. The Rochester Coronary Heart Disease Project: effect of cigarette smoking, hypertension, diabetes, and steroidal estrogen use on coronary heart disease among 40- to 59-year-old women, 1960 through 1982. *Mayo Clinic Proceedings* 64:1471, 1989.

Bergmann S, Siegert G, Wahrburg U, Schulte H, Assmann G, Jaros W, Drecan Team. Influence of menopause and lifestyle factors on high density lipoproteins in middle-aged women. *Journal of the North American Menopause Society* 4:52, 1997.

Chen FP, Lee N, Soong YK. Changes in the lipoprotein profile in postmenopausal women receiving hormone replacement therapy: effects of natural and synthetic progesterone. *Journal of Reproductive Medicine* 43:568, 1998

Clarkson TB, Shivley CA, Morgan TM, et al. Oral contraceptives and coronary artery atherosclerosis of cynomolgus monkeys. *Obstetrics Gynecology* 75:217, 1990.

Collins P, Rosano MC, Sarrel PM, et al. 17-beta estradiol attenuates acetylcholine-induced coronary arterial constriction in women but not men with coronary heart disease. *Circulation* 92:24, 1995.

Comp PC. Thrombophlebitis and pulmonary embolism in menopausal women. *Menopause* 5:2, 1997.

Crook D, Cust MP, Gangar KF, et al. Comparison of transdermal and oral estrogen-progestin replacement therapy: effects on serum lipids and lipoproteins. *The American Journal of Obstetrics and Gynecology* 166:950, 1992.

Daly E, Vessey M, Hawkins M, et al. Risk of venous thromboembolism in users of hormone replacement therapy. *Lancet* 348:977, 1996.

Falkeborn M, Persson I, Terent A, et al. Hormone replacement therapy and risk of stroke follow-up of a population-based cohort in Sweden. *Archives of Internal Medicine* 153:1201, 1993.

Ganz P, Gerhard M. How do we explain the clinical benefits of estrogen? From bedside to bench. (Editorial) *Circulation* 92:5, 1995.

Gilligan DM, Quyyume AA, Cannon RO. Effects of physiological levels of estrogen on coronary vasomotor function in postmenopausal women. *Circulation* 89:2545, 1994.

Gordon F, Kannel WB, Hjortland MC, McNamara PM. Menopause and coronary heart disease: the Framingham Study. *Annals of Internal Medicine* 89:157, 1978.

Grady D, Rubin SM, Petitti DB, et al. Hormone therapy to prevent disease and prolong life in postmenopausal women. *Annals of Internal Medicine* 117:1016, 1992.

Grodstein F, Stampfer MJ. The epidemiology of coronary heart disease and estrogen replacement in postmenopausal women. *Progress in Cardiovascular Diseases* 18:199, 1995.

Grodstein F, Stampfer M, Goldhaber S, et al. Prospective study of exogenous hormones and risk of pulmonary embolism in women. *Lancet* 348:983, 1996.

Gruchow HW, Anderson AJ, Barboriak JJ, Sobocinski KA. Postmenopausal use of estrogen and occlusion of coronary arteries. *American Heart Journal* 115:954, 1988.

Hassager C, Christiansen C. Blood pressure during oestrogen/progestogen substitution therapy in healthy postmenopausal women. *Maturitas* 9:315, 1988.

Henderson BE, Paganini-Hill A, Ross RK. Estrogen replacement and protection from acute myocardial infarction. *American Journal of Obstetrics and Gynecology* 159:312, 1998.

Henderson BE, Paganini-Hill A, Rose RK. Decreased mortality in users of estrogen replacement therapy. *Archives of Internal Medicine* 151:75, 1991.

Henderson BE, Ross RK, Paganini-Hill A. Estrogen use and cardiovascular disease. *American Journal of Obstetrics and Gynecology* 154:1181, 1986.

Hong MK, Romm PA, Reagan K, Green CE, Rackley CE. Effects of estrogen replacement therapy on serum lipid values and angiographically defined coronary artery disease in postmenopausal women. *American Journal of Cardiology* 69:176, 1992.

Jick H, Derby L, Myers M, Vasilakis C, Newton K. Risk of hospital admission for idiopathic venous thromboembolism among users of postmenopausal oestrogens. *Lancet* 348:981, 1996.

Kannel WB. Metabolic risk factors for coronary heart disease in women: perspective from the Framingham Study. *American Heart Journal* 114:413, 1987.

Koh KK, Mincemoyer R, Bui MN, et al. Efforts of hormone-replacement therapy on fibrinolysis in postmenopausal women. *New England Journal of Medicine* 336:683, 1997.

The Lipid Research Clinics Program. The lipid research clinics coronary primary prevention trial results. I: Reduction of incidence of coronary heart disease. *Journal of the American Medical Association* 251:351, 1984.

Lisbona H, Gorodeski GI, Utian WH. The role of platelets in prevention of coronary heart disease in postmenopausal women: a review. *Journal of the North American Menopause Society* 1:227, 1994.

McDonald CC, Stewart HG. Fatal myocardial infarction in the Scottish adjuvant tamoxifen trial. *British Medical Journal* 303:435, 1991.

McFarland KF, Boniface ME, Hornung CA, Earnhardt W, Humphries JO. Risk factors and noncontraceptive estrogen use in women with and without coronary disease. *American Heart Journal* 117:1209, 1989.

Nabulsi AA, Folsom AR, White A, et al. Association of hormone replacement therapy with various cardiovascular risk factors in postmenopausal women. *New England Journal of Medicine* 328:1069, 1993.

Nachtigall LE, Nachtigall RH, Nachtigall RD, Beckman EM. Estrogen replacement therapy II: a prospective study in the relationship to carcinoma and cardiovascular and metabolic problems. *Obstetrics Gynecology* 54:74, 1979.

Nasr A, Breckwoldt M. Estrogen replacement therapy and cardiovascular protection: lipid mechanisms are the tip of an iceberg. *Gynecology Endocrinology* 12:43, 1998.

Newman KP, Sullivan JM. Coronary heart disease in women: epidemiology clinical syndromes and management. *Journal of the North American Menopause Society* 3:51, 1996.

O'Keefe JF, Kim SC, Hall RR, et al. Estrogen replacement therapy after coronary angioplasty in women. *Journal of the American College of Cardiology* 29:1, 1997.

Ottosson UB, Johansson BG, von Schoultz B. Subfractions of high-density lipoprotein cholesterol during estrogen replacement therapy: a comparison between progestogens and natural progesterone. *The American Journal of Obstetrics and Gynecology* 151:746, 1985.

Paganini-Hill A. Estrogen replacement therapy and stroke. *Progress in Cardiovascular Disease* 38:223, 1995.

Paganini-Hill A, Ross RK, Henderson BE. Postmenopausal oestrogen treatment and stroke: a prospective study. *British Medical Journal* 297:51–59, 1988.

Perlman J, Wolf P, Finucane F, Madans J. Menopause and the epidemiology of cardiovascular disease in women. *Progress in Clinical Biological Research* 320:283, 1989.

Petitti DB, Wingerd J, Pellgrin F, Ramcharan S. Risk of vascular disease in women: smoking, oral contraceptives, non-contraceptive estrogens and other factors. *Journal of the American Medical Association* 242:1150, 1979.

Penotti M, Farina M, Sirone L, et al. Long-term effects of postmenopausal hormone replacement therapy on pulsatility index of internal carotid and middle cerebral arteries. *Journal of the North American Menopause Society* 4:101, 1997.

Pfeffer RI, Kurasaki TT, Charlton SK. Estrogen use and blood pressure in later life. *American Journal of Epidemiology* 110:469, 1979.

Pines A, Fishman EZ, Levo Y, et al. The effects of hormone replacement therapy in normal postmenopausal women: measurements of Doppler-derived parameters of aortic flow. *American Journal of Obstetrics and Gynecology* 164:806, 1991.

Ross RK, Pike MC, Henderson BE, Mack TM, Lobo RA. Stroke prevention and oestrogen replacement therapy. (Letter) *Lancet* 1:505, 1989.

Sands RH, Studd JWW, Crook D, et al. The effect of estrogen on blood pressure in hypertensive postmenopausal women. *Journal of the North American Menopause Society* 4:115, 1997.

Sarrel PM. How progestins compromise the cardioprotective effects of estrogens. (Editorial) *Journal of the North American Menopause Society* 2:187, 1995.

Shemesh J, Frexzel Y, Leibovitch L, et al. Does hormone replacement therapy inhibit coronary artery calcification? *Obstetrics Gynecology* 89:989, 1997.

Sherwin BB, Gelfand MM. A prospective one-year study of estrogen and progestin in postmenopausal women: effects on clinical symptoms and lipoprotein lipids. *Obstetrics Gynecology* 73:759, 1989.

Soler JT, Folsom AR, Kaye SA, Prineasa RJ. Association of abdominal adiposity, fasting insulin, sex hormone binding globulin and estrogen with lipids and lipoproteins in postmenopausal women. *Atherosclerosis* 79:21, 1989.

Speroff T, Dawson NV, Speroff L, Harber RJ. A risk-benefit analysis of elective bilateral oophorectomy: effects of changes in compliance with estrogen therapy an outcome. *American Journal of Obstetrics and Gynecology* 164:165, 1991.

Stampfer MJ, Colditz GA. Estrogen replacement therapy and coronary heart disease: a quantitative assessment of the epidemiological evidence. *Preventive Medicine* 20:47, 1991.

Stampfer MJ, Colditz GA, Willett WC. A prospective of postmenopausal estrogen therapy and coronary heart disease. *New England Journal of Medicine* 313:1044, 1985.

Stampfer MJ, Colditz GA, Willett WC, et al. Postmenopausal estrogen and cardiovascular disease: ten-year follow-up from the Nurses Health Study. *New England Journal of Medicine* 325:756, 1991.

Stampfer MJ, Krauss RH, Ma J. A prospective study of triglyceride level, low-density lipoprotein particle diameter and risk of myocardial infarction. *Journal of the American Medical Association* 276:882, 1996.

Sullivan JM, Fowlkes LP. The clinical aspects of estrogen and the cardiovascular system. *Obstetrics Gynecology* 87(Suppl):36S, 1996.

Sullivan JM, Shala BA, Miller LA, Lerner JL, McBrayer JO. Progestin enhances vasoconstrictor responses in postmenopausal women receiving estrogen replacement therapy. *Journal of the North American Menopause Society* 2:193, 1995.

Sullivan JM, Vander Zwaag R, Hughes JP, et al. Estrogen replacement and coronary artery disease: effect on survival in postmenopausal women. *Archives of Internal Medicine* 150:2557, 1990.

Sullivan JM, Vander Zwaag R, Lemp GF, et al. Postmenopausal estrogen use and coronary atherosclerosis. *Annals of Internal Medicine* 108:358, 1988.

The Writing Group for the PEPI Trial. Effects of estrogen or estrogen/progestin regimens on heart disease risk factors in postmenopausal women: the Postmenopausal Estrogen/Progestin Interventions (PEPI) Trial. *Journal of the American Medical Association* 273:199, 1995.

Thompson SG, Meade TW, Greenberg G. The use of hormonal replacement therapy and the risk of stroke and myocardial infarction in women. *Journal of Epidemiology in Community Health* 43:173, 1989.

Tucker ME. ERT may reduce risk of developing type 2 diabetes: estrogen also seems to improve blood sugar control in women who have diabetes. *Obstetric/Gynecologic News*. July 15, 1998.

Wenger NG. Coronary heart disease in women. *Haymarket Dogma*, New York, 1987, pp 122.

Wenger NK, Speroff L, Packard S. Cardiovascular health and disease in women. *New England Journal of Medicine* 329:247, 1993.

Wild R. The importance of LDL oxidation. (Editorial) *Journal of the North American Menopause Society* 4:191, 1997.

Wild RA. Estrogen: effects on the cardiovascular tree. *Obstetrics Gynecology* 87(Suppl):27S, 1996.

Wild RA, Taylor EL, Knehans A. The gynecologist and the prevention of cardiovascular disease. *The American Journal of Obstetrics and Gynecology* 172:1, 1995.

Wild RA. Role of obstetrics/gynecology in cardiovascular disease. *Journal of the North American Menopause Society* 3:122, 1996.

Wolf PH, Madans JH, Finucane FF, Higgins M, Kleinman JC. Reduction of cardiovascular disease–related mortality among postmenopausal women who use hormones: evidence from a national cohort. *The American Journal of Obstetrics and Gynecology* 164:489, 1991.

Wren BG, Routledge AD. The effect of type and dose of oestrogen on the blood pressure of postmenopausal women. *Maturitas* 5:135, 1983.

Yeung AC, Vekshteise VI, Krantz DS. The effect of atherosclerosis on the vasomotor response of coronary arteries to mental stress. *New England Journal of Medicine* 325:1551, 1991.

CHAPTER 3
ESTROGEN AND THE BRAIN: MODERN WONDERS

Ballinger CB. Psychiatric aspects of the menopause. *British Journal of Psychiatry* 156:773, 1990.

Barrett-Connor E, Kritz-Silverstein D. Estrogen replacement therapy and cognitive function in older women. *Journal of the American Medical Association* 269:2637, 1993.

Cagnacci A, Volpe A, Arangino S, et al. Depression and anxiety in climacteric women: role of hormone replacement therapy. *Journal of the North American Menopause Society* 4:206, 1997.

Chatel A, Fugère P, Bissonnette F, Bérubé S. Psychological distress and sexuality in a group of women attending a menopause clinic: effect of hormonal replacement therapy. *Journal of the North American Menopause Society* 3:165, 1996.

Ditkoff EC, Crary WG, Cristo M, Lobo RA. Estrogen improves psychological function in asymptomatic postmenopausal women. *Obstetrics Gynecology* 78:991, 1991.

Falheborn M, Persson I, Terént A, et al. Hormone replacement therapy and the risk of stroke. *Archives of Internal Medicine* 153:1201, 1993.

Flöter A, Nathorst-Böös J, Carlström K, Von Schoultz B. Androgen status and sexual life in perimenopausal women. *Journal of the North American Menopause Society* 4:95, 1997.

Gassman A, Santoro N. The influence of menopausal hormone changes on sexuality: current knowledge and recommendations for practice. *Journal of the North American Menopause Society* 1:91, 1994.

Hammar ML, Lindgreen R, Berg GE, Möller CG, Niklasson MK. Effects of hormonal replacement therapy on the postural balance among postmenopausal women. *Obstetrics Gynecology* 88:955, 1996.

Henderson V. The epidemiology of estrogen replacement therapy and Alzheimer's disease. *Neurology* 48(Suppl 7):S27, 1997.

Kampex DL, Sherwin BB. Estrogen use and verbal memory in healthy postmenopausal women. *Obstetrics Gynecology* 83:979, 1994.

Kanas C, Resnick S, Morrison A, et al. A prospective study of estrogen replacement therapy and the risk of developing Alzheimer's disease: the Baltimore Longitudinal Study of Aging. *Neurology* 48:1517, 1997.

Limouzin-Lamothe MA, Mairon N, Joyce CRB, LeGal M. Quality of life after the menopause: influence of hormonal replacement therapy. *American Journal of Obstetrics and Gynecology* 170:618, 1994.

Maoz B, Shiber A, Lazer S, Lopernik G. The prevalence of psychological distress among postmenopausal women attending a menopausal clinic and the effect of hormone replacement therapy on their mental state. *Journal of the North American Menopause Society* 1:137, 1994.

Naessen T, Lindmark B, Larsen HC. Better postural balance in elderly women receiving estrogens. *The American Journal of Obstetrics and Gynecology* 177:412, 1997.

Ohkura T, Teshima Y, Isse K. Estrogen increases cerebral and cerebellar blood flow in postmenopausal women. *Journal of the North American Menopause Society* 2:13, 1995.

Paganini-Hill A. Alzheimer's disease in women: Can estrogen play a preventive role? *The Female Patient* 23:12, 1998 (March).

Paganini-Hill A, Henderson VW. Estrogen replacement therapy and risk of Alzheimer's disease. *Archives of Internal Medicine* 156:2213, 1996.

Palinkas LA, Barrett-Connor F. Estrogen use and depressive symptoms in postmenopausal women. *Obstetrics Gynecology* 80:30, 1992.

Pearlstein JB. Hormones and depression: What are the facts about premenstrual syndrome, menopause and hormone replacement therapy? *The American Journal of Obstetrics and Gynecology* 173:646, 1995.

Phillips SM, Sherwin BB. Effects of estrogen on memory function in surgically menopausal women. *Psychoneuroendocrinology* 17:485, 1992.

Schiff I, Registein Q, Tulchinksy D, Ryan KJ. Effects of estrogens on sleep and psychological state of hypogonadal women. *Journal of the American Medical Association* 242:2405, 1979.

Schneider LS, Farlow MR, Henderson VW, Pogoda JM. Effects of estrogen replacement therapy on response to tacrine in patients with Alzheimer's disease. *Neurology* 46:1580, 1996.

Sherwin BB. Affective changes with estrogen and androgen replacement therapy in surgically menopausal women. *Journal of Affective Disorders* 14:177, 1988.

Sherwin BB. Estrogen, the brain, and memory. *Journal of the North American Menopause Society* 3:97, 1996.

Sherwin BB. Estrogen effects on cognition in menopausal women. *Neurology* 48(Suppl 7):S21, 1997.

Sherwin BB. Hormones, mood and cognitive functioning in postmenopausal women. *Obstetrics Gynecology* 87(Suppl 2):20S, 1996.

Sherwin BB, Gelfand MM. Sex steroids and effects in the surgical menopause: a double-blind, cross-over study. *Psychoneuroendocrinology* 10:325, 1985.

Tang MX, Jacobs, D, Stern Y, et al. Effect of oestrogen during menopause on risk and age at onset of Alzheimer's disease. *Lancet* 342:429, 1996.

Watts NB, Notelovitz M, Timmons MC, et al. Comparison of oral estrogens and estrogens plus androgen on bone mineral density, menopausal symptoms, and lipid-lipoprotein profiles in surgical menopause. *Obstetrics Gynecology* 85:529, 1995.

Yaffe K, Saaya G, Liebeburg I, Grady D. Estrogen therapy in postmenopausal women: effects on cognitive function and dementia. *Journal of the American Medical Association* 279:688, 1998.

CHAPTER 4
ESTROGEN PREVENTS BONE LOSS

Archer DF. Is there an effect of progestin or progesterone on bone mineral density? (Editorial) *Journal of the North American Menopause Society* 3:3, 1996.

Cauley JA, Lucas FL, Kuller LH, et al. Bone mineral density and risk of breast cancer in older women: the study of osteoporotic fractures. *Journal of the American Medical Association* 276:1404, 1996.

Cauley JA, Seeley DG, Ensrud K, et al. Estrogen replacement therapy and fractures in older women. *Annals of Internal Medicine* 122:9, 1995.

Chapuy MC, Arlot ME, Duboeuf F, et al. Vitamin D3 and calcium to prevent hip fractures in elderly women. *New England Journal of Medicine* 327:1637, 1992.

Chestnut CH III. The role of bone resorption markers in managing menopausal women on HRT. *OBG Management* (Suppl) 6, October 1997.

Christiansen C, Nilas L, Riis BJ, Rodbro P, Deftos L. Uncoupling of bone formation and resorption by combined oestrogen and progestogen therapy in postmenopausal osteoporosis. *Lancet* 2:800, 1985.

Consensus Development Conference. Diagnosis, prophylaxis, and treatment of osteoporosis. *American Journal of Medicine* 94:64, 1993.

Cummings SR, Black DM, Nevitt MC, et al. Bone density at various sites for prediction of hip fractures. *Lancet* 341:72, 1993.

DeSouza MJ, Prestwood KM, Luciano AA, Miller BE, Nulsen JC. A comparison of the effect of synthetic and micronized hormone replacement therapy on bone mineral density and biochemical markers of bone metabolism. *Journal of the North American Menopause Society* 3:140, 1996.

Ebeling P, Atley L, Guthrie JR, et al. Bone turnover markers and bone density across the menopausal transition. *Journal of Clinical Endocrinology and Metabolism* 81:3366, 1996.

Ettinger B. Prevention of osteoporosis: treatment of estradiol deficiency. *Obstetrics Gynecology* 72:125, 1988.

Ettinger B, Genant HK, Cann CE. Postmenopausal bone loss is prevented by treatment with low-dosage estrogen with calcium. *Annals of Internal Medicine* 106:40, 1987.

Ettinger B, Genant HK, Cann CE. Long-term estrogen replacement therapy prevents bone loss and fractures. *Annals of Internal Medicine* 102:319, 1985.

Ettinger B, Genant HK, Steiger P, Madvig P. Low-dosage micronized 17B-estradiol prevents bone loss in postmenopausal women. *The American Journal of Obstetrics and Gynecology* 166:479, 1992.

Eyre DR. How biochemical markers measure bone remodeling activity. *OBG Management* (Suppl) 3, October 1997.

Felson DT, Zhang Y, Hannan MT, et al. The effect of postmenopausal estrogen therapy on bone density in elderly women. *New England Journal of Medicine* 329:1141, 1993.

Gass MLS. Osteoporosis and the gynecologist: a call for action. *Contemporary Obstetrics and Gynecology* 58, Nov 1997.

Holt LH, Taft LB, Moulthrop JM. Bone density measurement: survey of use and impact on treatment. *Journal of the North American Menopause Society* 4:219, 1997.

Horowitz M. Cytokines and estrogen in bone: antiosteoporotic effects. *Science* 260:626, 1993.

Jensen J, Christiansen C, Rodbro P. Cigarette smoking, serum estrogens, and bone loss during hormone replacement therapy early after menopause. *New England Journal of Medicine* 313:973, 1985.

Johnson CC Jr., Slemenda CW, Melton LJ III. Clinical use of bone densitometry. *New England Journal of Medicine* 324:1105, 1991.

Kiel DP, Felson DT, Anderson JJ, Wilson PWF, Moskowitz MA. Hip fracture and the use of estrogen in postmenopausal women: the Framingham Study. *New England Journal of Medicine* 317:1169, 1987.

Lafferty FW, Fiske ME. Postmenopausal estrogen replacement: a long-term cohort study. *American Journal of Medicine* 97:66, 1994.

Lees B, Molleson T, Arnett TR, Stevenson JC. Differences in proximal femur bone density over two centuries. *Lancet* 341:673, 1993.

Lindsay R. The menopause and osteoporosis. *Obstetrics Gynecology* 87(Suppl):17S, 1996.

Lindsay R. Prevention and treatment of osteoporosis. *Lancet* 341:801, 1993.

Lindsay R, Hart DM, Clark DM. The minimum effective dose of estrogen for postmenopausal bone loss. *Obstetrics Gynecology* 63:759, 1984.

Lindsay R, MacLean A, Kraszewski A, Clark AC, Garwood J. Bone response to termination of estrogen treatment. *Lancet* 1:1325, 1978.

Lufkin EG, Wahner HW, O'Fallon WM, et al. Treatment of postmenopausal osteoporosis with transdermal estrogen. *Annals of Internal Medicine* 117:1, 1992.

McKane RW, Khosla S, Ristell J, et al. Role of estrogen deficiency in pathogenesis of secondary hyperparathyroidism and increased bone resorption in elderly women. *Proceedings of the Association of American Physicians* 109:174, 1997.

Munk-Jensen N, Nielsen SP, Obel EB, Eriksin PB. Reversal of postmenopausal vertebral bone loss by oestrogen and progestogen: a double blind placebo controlled study. *British Medical Journal* 296:1150, 1988.

Munk-Jensen N, Overgaard K, Nilas L. Postmenopausal bone loss and response to hormone replacement therapy independent of climacteric symptoms. *Journal of the North American Menopause Society* 2:35, 1995.

Naessén T, Persson I, Thor L, et al. Maintained bone density at advanced ages after long-term treatment with low dose estradiol implants. *British Journal of Obstetrics and Gynecology* 100:454, 1993.

Ooms ME, Ross JC, Benzener PD, et al. Prevention of bone loss by vitamin D supplementation in elderly women: a randomized double blind trial. *Journal of Clinical Endocrinology and Metabolism* 80:1052, 1995.

Paganini Hill A, Chao A, Ross RK, Henderson BE. Exercise and other factors in prevention of hip fracture. The Leisure World Study. *Epidemiology* 2:16, 191.

Panay N, Studd J. Do progestogens and progesterone reduce bone loss? *Journal of the North American Menopause Society* 3:13, 1996.

Prince RL, Smith M, Dick IM, et al. Prevention of postmenopausal osteoporosis: a comparative study of exercise, calcium supplementation, and hormone-replacement therapy. *New England Journal of Medicine* 325:1189, 1991.

Prockop DJ. The genetic trail of osteoporosis. (Editorial) *New England Journal of Medicine* 338:1061, 1998.

Quigley MET, Martin PL, Burnier AM, Brooks P. Estrogen therapy arrests bone loss in elderly women. *American Journal of Obstetrics and Gynecology* 156:1516, 1987.

Reid IR, Ames RW, Evans MC, Gamble GD, Sharpe JS. Effect of calcium supplementation on bone loss in postmenopausal women. *New England Journal of Medicine* 328:460, 1993.

Riis BJ. Biochemical markers of bone turnover II: diagnosis, prophylaxis, and treatment of osteoporosis. *American Journal of Medicine* 95 (Suppl 5A):17S, 1993.

Seeman E, Hopper JL, Bach LI, et al. Reduced bone mass in daughters of women with osteoporosis. *New England Journal of Medicine* 320:554, 1989.

Silverman SL, Greenwald M, Klein RA, Drinkwater BL. Effect of bone density information on decisions about hormone replacement therapy: a randomized trial. *Obstetrics Gynecology* 89:321, 1997.

Stevenson JC, Cust MP, Gangar KF, et al. Effects of transdermal versus oral hormone replacement therapy on bone density in spine and proximal femur in postmenopausal women. *Lancet* 336:1327, 1990.

Uitterlinden SG, Burger H, Huang Q, et al. Relation of alleles of the collagen Type I gene to bone density and the risk of osteoporotic fractures in postmenopausal women. *New England Journal of Medicine* 338:1016, 1998.

Vergnaud P, Garnero P, Meunier PJ, et al. Undercarboxylated osteocalcin measured with a specific immunoassay predicts hip fracture in elderly women: the EPIDOS Study. *Journal of Clinical Endocrinology and Metabolism* 82:719, 1997.

Weiss NC, Ure CL, Ballard JH, Williams AR, Dalixg JR. Estimated incidence of fractures of the lower forearm and hip in postmenopausal women. *New England Journal of Medicine* 303:1195, 1980.

The Writing Group for the PEPI Trial. Effects of hormone therapy on bone mineral density: results from the Postmenopausal Estrogen/Progestin (PEPI) Trial. *Journal of the American Medical Association* 276:1389, 1996.

CHAPTER 5
HORMONE REPLACEMENT DOES NOT CAUSE UTERINE CANCER

Baker DD. Estrogen in patients with previous endometrial carcinoma. *Comprehensive Therapy* 16:28, 1990.

Botsis D, Kassanos D, Pyrgiotis E, Zourias PA. Vagina sonography of the endometrium in postmenopausal women. *Clinical and Experimental Obstetrics and Gynecology* 19:189, 1992.

Brinton LA, Hoover RN, and the Endometrial Cancer Collaborative Group. Estrogen replacement therapy and endometrial cancer risk. *Unresolved Issues* 81:265, 1993.

Chapman JA, DiSaia PJ, Osann K, et al. Estrogen replacement in surgical stage I and II endometrial cancer survivors. *The American Journal of Obstetrics and Gynecology* 175:1995.

Comerci JT, Fields AL, Runowicz CD, Goldberg GL. Continuous low-dose combined hormone replacement therapy and the risk of endometrial cancer. *Gynecologic Oncology* 64:425, 1997.

Creasman WT. Estrogen replacement therapy: Is previously treated cancer a contraindication? *Obstetrics Gynecology* 77:308, 1991.

Cushing KL, Weiss NS, Voight LF, McKnight B, Beresford SAA. Risk of endometrial cancer in relation to use of low-dose, unopposed estrogens. *Obstetrics Gynecology* 91:35, 1998.

Grady D, Gebretsadik T, Kerlikowski K, Ernster V, Petitti D. Hormone replacement therapy and endometrial cancer risk: a meta-analysis. *Obstetrics Gynecology* 85:304, 1995.

Hempling RE, Wong C, Piver MS, Natarajan N, Mettlin CJ. Hormone replacement therapy as a risk factor for epithelial ovarian cancer: results of a case-control study. *Obstetrics Gynecology* 89:1012, 1997.

Lee RB, Burke TW, Park RC. Estrogen replacement therapy following treatment for Stage I endometrial carcinoma. *Gynecologic Oncology* 36:189, 1990.

Pansini F, DePaoli D, Serra MM. Combined use of progesterone challenge test and endometrium challenge test and endometrium thickness evaluated by transvaginal ultrasonography in the preventive management of postmenopausal women. *Gynecologic and Obstetric Investigation* 34:237, 1992.

Persson I, Yuen J, Berkgvist, Schairer C. Cancer incidence and mortality in receiving estrogen and estrogen replacement therapy long-term follow-up of a Swedish cohort. *International Journal of Cancer* 67:327, 1996.

Pickar JH, Thorneycroft I, Whitehead M. Effects of hormone replacement therapy on the endometrium and lipid parameters: a review of randomized clinical trials, 1985 to 1995. *American Journal of Obstetrics and Gynecology* 178:1087, 1998.

Weiss NS, Beresford SAA, Voigt LF, McKnight B. Estrogen-progestin replacement therapy and endometrial cancer. *Journal of the National Cancer Institute* 90:164, 1998.

Wolfe BMJ, Koval JJ, Niskar JA. Effects of adding C-19 versus C-21 progestin to conjugated estrogen in moderately hypercholesterolemic postmenopausal women. *American Journal of Obstetrics and Gynecology* 278:787, 1998.

Woodruff JD, Pickar JH. Incidence of endometrial hyperplasia in postmenopausal women taking conjugated estrogens (Premarin) with Medroxyprogesterone acetate or conjugated estrogens alone. *American Journal of Obstetrics and Gynecology* 170:1213, 1994.

CHAPTER 6
THE PERKS: HOW ESTROGEN IMPROVES THE QUALITY OF LIFE

Aksel S, Schomberg DW, Tyrey L, Hammond CB. Vasomotor symptoms, serum estrogens and gonadotropin levels in surgical menopause. *American Journal of Obstetrics and Gynecology* 126:165, 1976.

Barbarch L. Loss of sexual desire. *Menopause Management* 7:10, 1998.

Bhatia NN, Bergman A, Karram MM. Effects of estrogen on urethral function in woman with urinary incontinence. *Obstetrics Gynecology* 160:176, 1989.

Castelo-Branco C, Duran M, Gonzalez-Merlo J. Skin collagen changes related to age and hormone replacement therapy. *Maturitas* 15:113, 1992.

Daniell HW. Postmenopausal tooth loss: contributions to edentulism by osteoporosis and cigarette smoking. *Archives of Internal Medicine* 143:1679, 1993.

Fantl JA, Bump RC, Robinson D, McClish DK, Wyman JF, and the Continence Program for Women Research Group. Efficacy of estrogen supplementation in the treatment of urinary incontinence. *Obstetrics Gynecology* 88:745, 1996.

Grodstein F, Martinez E, Platz EA, et al. Postmenopausal hormone use and risk for colorectal cancer and adenoma. *Annals of Internal Medicine* 128:705, 1998.

Haarbs J, Marslew U, Gotfredsen A, Christiansen C. Postmenopausal hormone replacement therapy central distribution of body fat after menopause. *Metabolism* 40:1323, 1991.

Hardiman P, Ginsburg J. Vascular effects of veralipride, a non-hormonal treatment for climacteric flushing. *Journal of the North American Menopause Society* 2:219, 1995.

Kronenberg F. Hot flashes: epidemiology and physiology. *Annals of the New York Academy of Science* 592:52, 1990.

Ley CJ, Lees B, Stevenson JC. Sex and menopause-associated changes in body-fat distribution. *American Journal of Clinical Nutrition* 55:950, 1992.

Lusto R, Männistö S, Vartiainen F. Hormone replacement therapy and body size: How much does lifestyle explain? *American Journal of Obstetrics and Gynecology* 178:66, 1998.

Maheux R, Naud F, Rioux M, et al. A randomized double-blind, placebo-controlled study on the effect of conjugated estrogens on skin thickness. *American Journal of Obstetrics and Gynecology* 170:642, 1994.

Nevitt MC, Cummings SR, Lane NE, et al. Association of estrogen replacement therapy with the risk of osteoarthritis of the hip in elderly white women. *Archives of Internal Medicine* 156:2073, 1996.

Oliveria SA, Felson OT, Klein RA, Reed JI, Walker AM. Estrogen replacement therapy and the development of osteoarthritis. *Epidemiology* 7:415, 1996.

Oliveria SA, Klein RA, Reed JI, et al. Estrogen replacement therapy and urinary tract infections in postmenopausal women aged 45–89. *Journal of the North American Menopause Society* 5:4, 1998.

Polo-Kantola P, Erkkola R, Helenius H, Irjala K, Polo O. When does replacement therapy improve sleep quality? *American Journal of Obstetrics and Gynecology* 178:1002, 1998.

Schiff I, Regestein Q, Tulchinsky D, Ryan KJ. Effects of estrogens on sleep and psychological state of hypogonadal women. *Journal of the American Medical Association* 242:2405, 1979.

Sherwin BB. Affective changes with estrogen and androgen replacement therapy in surgically menopausal women. *Journal of Affective Disorders* 14:177, 1988.

Sherwin BB. The impact of different doses of estrogen and progestin on mood and sexual behaviour in postmenopausal women. *Journal of Clinical Endocrinology and Metabolism* 72:336, 1991.

Sherwin BB, Gelfand MM. Sex steroids and effect in the surgical menopause: a double-blind, cross-over study. *Psychoneuroendocrinology* 10:325, 1985.

Vandenbruocke JP, Witteman JCM, Valkenburg HA, et al. Noncontraceptive hormones and rheumatoid arthritis in perimenopausal and postmenopausal women. *Journal of the American Medical Association* 255:1299, 1986.

Versi E, Cardozo L, Studd J, Brincat M, Cooper D. Urinary disorders and the menopause. *Journal of the North American Menopause Society* 2:89, 1995.

Wingate L, Wingate MB, Hassanein S. The relation between overweight and urinary incontinence in postmenopausal women: a case control study. *Journal of the North American Menopause Society* 1:199, 1994.

CHAPTER 7
HORMONE REGIMENS AND SIDE EFFECTS: AN OVERVIEW

Archer DF, Pickar JH, and Bottiglioni F, for The Menopause Group. Bleeding patterns in postmenopausal women taking continuous combined or sequential regiments of conjugated estrogens with medroxyprogesterone acetate. *Obstetrics Gynecology* 83:686, 1994.

Büyük E, Gürler A, Erenus M. Relationship between circulating estradiol levels, body mass index, and breakthrough bleeding in postmenopausal women receiving hormone replacement therapy. *Journal of the North American Menopause Society* 5:24, 1998.

Casper RF, Dodin S, Reid RL, and study investigators. The effect of 20 ug ethinyl estradiol/1 mg norethindrone acetate (Minestrin™), a low-dose oral contraceptive, on vaginal bleeding patterns, hot flashes, and quality of life in symptomatic perimenopausal women. *Journal of the North American Menopause Society* 4:139, 1997.

Cassidenti DL, Pike MC, Vyod AG, Stanczyk FZ, Lobo RA. A reevaluation of estrogen status in postmenopausal women who smoke. *American Journal of Obstetrics and Gynecology* 166:1444, 1992.

Ettinger B, Selby J, Citron JT, et al. Cyclic hormone replacement therapy using quarterly progestin. *Obstetrics Gynecology* 83:693, 1994.

Kessler CM, Szymanski LM, Shamsipour Z, et al. Estrogen replacement therapy and coagulation relationship to lipid and lipoprotein changes. *Obstetrics Gynecology* 89:326, 1997.

Lindheim SR, Notelovitz M, Feldman EB, et al. The independent effects of exercise and estrogen on lipids and lipoproteins in postmenopausal women. *Obstetrics Gynecology* 83:167, 1994.

Lobo RA. The role of progestins in hormone replacement therapy. *American Journal of Obstetrics and Gynecology* 166:1997, 1992.

Lobo RA, Pickar JH, Wild RA, Walsh B, Hirvonen E, for The Menopause Study Group. Metabolic impact of adding medroxyprogesterone acetate to conjugated estrogen therapy in postmenopausal women. *Obstetrics Gynecology* 84:989, 1994.

Nachtigall LE. Emerging delivery systems for estrogen replacement aspects of transdermal and oral delivery. *American Journal of Obstetrics and Gynecology* 173:993, 1995.

Nilsson K, Kumer G. Low-dose oestradiol in the treatment of urogenital oestrogen deficiency: a pharmacokinetic and pharmacodynamic study. *Maturitis* 15:121, 1992.

The North American Menopause Society. Achieving long-term continuance of menopausal ERT/HRT: consensus opinion of the North American Menopause Society. *Journal of the North American Menopause Society* 5:69, 1998.

Rigg LA, Hermann H, Yen SSC. Absorption of estrogens from vaginal creams. *New England Journal of Medicine* 298:195, 1978.

Rosenberg MJ, King TDN, Timmons MC. Estrogen androgen for hormone replacement: a review. *Journal of Reproductive Medicine* 42:394, 1997.

Shoupe D, Mishell DR. Contraindications to hormone replacement: treatment of the postmenopausal woman. *Basic and Clinical Aspects* 415, 1994.

Udoff L, Langenberg P, Adashi EY. Combined continuous hormone replacement therapy: a critical review. *Obstetrics Gynecology* 86:306, 1995.

Whitcroft SI, Crook D, Marsh MS, et al. Long-term effects of oral and transdermal hormone replacement therapies on serum lipid and lipoprotein concentrations. *Obstetrics Gynecology* 84:222, 1994.

Williams DB, Voight BJ, Fu YS, Schoenfeld MJ, Judd HL. Assessment of less than monthly progestin therapy in postmenopausal women given estrogen replacement. *Obstetrics Gynecology* 84:787, 1994.

CHAPTER 8
"DESIGNER" ESTROGENS: SCANDALOUS FOLLIES OF THE NINETIES

Adler S, Sadovsky Y. Selective modulation of estrogen receptor action. *Journal of Clinical Endocrinology and Metabolism* 83:3, 1998.

Berlière M, Charles A, Galant C, Donnez J. Uterine side of tamoxifen: a need for systematic pretreatment screening. *Obstetrics Gynecology* 91:40, 1998.

Burke W, LaCroix AZ. Breast cancer and hormone replacement therapy. *Lancet* 350:1042, 1997.

Chang J, Powles TJ, Ashley SE, Iveson T, Gregory RK, Dowsett M. Variation in endometrial thickening in women with amenorrhea on tamoxifen. *Breast Cancer Research and Treatment* 48:85, 1998.

Cheng WF, Lin HH, Torng PL, Huang SC. Comparison of endometrial changes among symptomatic tamoxifen-treated and nontreated premenopausal and postmenopausal breast cancer patients. *Gynecologic Oncology* 66:233, 1997.

Cohen I, Altaras MM, Beyth Y, et al. Estrogen and progesterone receptors in the endometrium of postmenopausal breast cancer patients treated with tamoxifen and progestogens. *Gynecologic Oncology* 65:83, 1997.

Cohen I, Rosen DJD, Shapira J, et al. Endometrial changes with tamoxifen: comparison between tamoxifen-treated and nontreated asymptomatic, postmenopausal breast cancer patients. *Gynecologic Oncology* 52:185, 1994.

Daniel Y, Inbar M, Bar-Am A, Peyser MR, Lessing JB. The effects of tamoxifen treatment on the endometrium. *Fertility-Sterility* 65:1083, 1996.

Delmas PD, Bjarnason NH, Mitlak BH, et al. Effects of raloxifene on bone mineral density, serum cholesterol concentrations, and uterine endometrium in postmenopausal women. *New England Journal of Medicine* 337:1641, 1997.

Fisher B, Costantino JP, Redmond CK, Fisher ER, Wickerman DL, Cronin WM, and other NSABP contributors. Endometrial cancer in tamoxifen-treated breast cancer patients: findings from the National Surgical Adjuvant Breast and Bowel Project (NSABP) B-14. *Journal of the National Cancer Institute* 86:527, 1994.

Gusberg SB. Tamoxifen for breast cancer associated endometrial cancer. *Cancer* April: 1464, 1990.

Heaney RP, Draper MW. Raloxifene and estrogen: comparative bone-remodeling kinetics. *Journal of Clinical Endocrinology and Metabolism* 82:3425, 1997.

Henig RM. Behind the buzz on designer estrogens, questions linger. *The New York Times,* Sunday, June 21, 1998.

Lahte E, Guillermo B, Kauppila A, et al. Endometrial changes in postmenopausal breast cancer patients receiving tamoxifen. *Obstetrics Gynecology* 81:660, 1993.

A menopause management roundtable discussion, SERMs in clinical practice: pieces of the puzzle. *Menopause Management,* 7, March–April 1998.

Nayfield SG, Gorin MB. Tamoxifen-associated eye disease: a review. *Journal of Clinical Oncology* 14:1018, 1996.

Neven P, Vergote I. Should tamoxifen users be screened for endometrial lesions? *Lancet* 351:155, 1998.

Penotti M, Sirone L, Miglierina L, et al. The effect of tamoxifen and transdermal 17B-estradiol on cerebral arterial vessels: a randomized controlled study. *American Journal of Obstetrics and Gynecology* 178:801, 1998.

Powles T, Eeles R, Ashley S, et al. Interim analysis of the incidence of breast cancer in the Royal Marsden Hospital tamoxifen randomised chemoprevention trial. *Lancet* 352:98, 1998.

Pritchard KI. Is tamoxifen effective in prevention of breast cancer? *Lancet* 352, 1998.

Rifkind BM, Rossouw JE. Of designer drugs, magic bullets and gold standards. (Editorial) *Journal of the American Medical Association* 279:1483, 1998.

Speroff L. Postmenopausal hormone therapy and breast cancer. Oregon Health Sciences University School of Medicine, 1997. *Contemporary Ob/Gyn,* Vol. 42, No. 1 (Suppl).

Speroff L. Postmenopausal hormone therapy and cardiovascular system. Oregon Health Sciences University School of Medicine, 1997. *Contemporary Ob/Gyn,* Vol. 42, No. 6 (Suppl).

Ugwunmadu AHN, Bower D, Ho PK. Tamoxifen induce adenomyosis and adenomyomatous endometrial polyp. *British Journal of Obstetrics and Gynecology* 100:396, 1993.

Van Leewven FE, Benraadt J, Coebergh JWW, et al. Risk of endometrial cancer after tamoxifen treatment of breast cancer. *Lancet* 343:448, 1994.

Veronese U, Maisonneuve P, Costa A, et al. On behalf of the Italian Tamoxifen Prevention Study. *Lancet* 352:93, 1998.

Walsh BW, Kuller LH, Wild RA, et al. Effects of raloxifene on serum lipids and coagulation factors in healthy postmenopausal women. *Journal of the American Medical Association* 279:1445, 1998.

Weiss NS, Beresford SAA, Voigt LF, McKnight B. Estrogen-progestin replacement therapy and endometrial cancer. *Journal of the National Cancer Institute* 90:164, 1998.

Yang NN, Venugopalan M, Hardikar S, Glasebrook A. Identification of an estrogen response element activated by metabolites of 17B-estradiol and raloxifene. *Science* 273:122, 1996.

APPENDIX A
SAVING LIVES WITH ESTROGEN: A LOOK AT THE NUMBERS

Gorsky RD, Koplan JP, Peterson HB, Thacker SB. Relative risks and benefits of long-term estrogen replacement therapy: a decision analysis. *Obstetrics Gynecology* 83:161, 1994.

Henderson BE, Paganini-Hill A, Ross RK. Decreased mortality in users of estrogen replacement therapy. *Archives of Internal Medicine* 151:75, 1991.

Henderson BE, Ross RK, Paganini-Hill A, Mack TM. Estrogen use and cardiovascular disease. *American Journal of Obstetrics and Gynecology* 154:1181, 1986.

Lobo R. Benefits and risks of estrogen replacement therapy. *American Journal of Obstetrics and Gynecology* 173:982, 1995.

U.S. Bureau of the Census. Projections of the population of the United States: 1977 to 2050. Current Population Reports, Series P-25, No. 704.

ACKNOWLEDGMENTS

I have been extremely lucky. At every turn I have been surrounded by people of talent and accomplishment. My earliest memories include a reverence for the musical genius, intelligence, and humor that characterized my parents and family. Later, I was fortunate enough to study under Hugh R. K. Barber, M.D., whose clinical, surgical, and academic genius are without peer. Anyone familiar with the irreverent wit of his editorials in the journal *The Female Patient,* as well as his abiding love for the practice and teaching of medicine, will instantly recognize from whom I draw inspiration.

Growing up with me under the tutelage of Dr. Barber was my forever friend and partner, Dr. Suzanne Yale—the only physician I know whose artful and brilliant practice of medicine can also be described as elegant. How truly lucky I am to have shared my career with her.

I have also had the loyal support of the very best nursing and office staff: Liz Pennisi, Sherry Sofsky, Marie Albanese, and Johanna Olsson.

In my fledgling career as a writer, I am indebted to my editor, Laura Yorke, who not only lent her remarkable talents to this effort, but also recognized its mission from the inception. My agent Kim Witherspoon matched me with my coauthor, Ina Yalof, for which I will always be grateful. Ina has brought to our collaboration many of the things I treasure—easy brilliance, a keen wit, and a particular affinity for a well-turned phrase. Her devotion to medicine and the care of others only strengthens our bond and reinforces the integrity of our relationship. Ina, Laura, and I will be forever linked by this shared endeavor to better women's lives.

In the preparation of this manuscript, I enjoyed the considerable talents of my typist, Elizabeth Armour, and my research assistant, Valerie Vasquez. Both were absolutely wonderful to work with.

Above all, these efforts would not have been possible without the lifelong support of my wife, Vivien, the love of my life.

INDEX

ABOUT THE AUTHORS

ADAM ROMOFF, M.D., is in private practice and is the Associate Director of Obstetrics and Gynecology at Lenox Hill Hospital in New York City, where he has been the Director of Resident Education for many years. He lives with his wife, Vivien, their three children, David, Peter, and Sarah, in Rye, New York.

INA YALOF is a medical sociologist and the author of *Open Heart Surgery: A Guidebook for Patients and Families*; *Life and Death: The Story of a Hospital*; and coauthor of *The Massachusetts General Hospital Book on Breast Cancer*. Her most recent book is *Straight from the Heart: Letters of Hope and Inspiration from Survivors of Breast Cancer*. She lives with her husband, Herbert, in Quincy, Massachusetts.